CHANT OF PLEASANT EXPLORATION

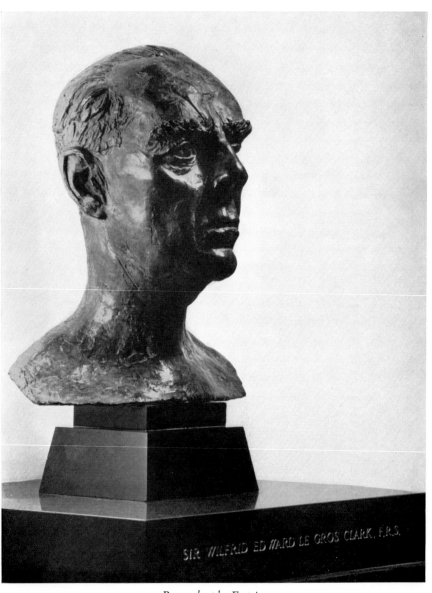

Bronze bust by Epstein

CHANT OF
PLEASANT
EXPLORATION

WILFRID LE GROS CLARK F.R.S.

E. & S. LIVINGSTONE LTD
EDINBURGH AND LONDON
1968

E. & S. LIVINGSTONE LTD

1968

SBN 443 00602 4

PRINTED IN GREAT BRITAIN

PREFACE

Autobiographies, it has been suggested, are little more than phantasies of memory. In a sense I suppose there may be a modicum of truth in such a cynicism. Of course, dates, names of places, sequences of events and so forth, can be faithfully recorded. But our evaluation of incidents that we have experienced and of personalities we have encountered in the past always tends later to be coloured by the richer insight that grows with advancing years. This must be so, but it does not necessarily follow that our memories are at fault. On the contrary.

I call to mind 'An Essay on Aesthetics' by that very readable art critic, Roger Fry, in which he remarks that 'man has the peculiar faculty of calling up in his mind an echo of past experiences . . . of going over it again, "in imagination" as we say'. He then goes on to make the point that in actual life we concentrate our attention on the practical needs of the moment and it is towards these that we bend our whole conscious endeavour. But in retrospection no such action is necessary, and in some ways we can thus contemplate an event more clearly simply because our attention is not distracted by immediate physical reactions and requirements. In other words, when we have a job to do, we are focussing our attention on doing it and considering how to complete it, to the extent that we do not consciously perceive details that for the moment seem irrelevant. Roger Fry was referring to the ability of the artist to render pictorially true relationships and harmonies of the perceptual world and to express in visual form the concomitant emotions which they arouse in his mind. This line of thought may equally well apply to reminiscences of past experiences expressed in writing, provided due care is taken to

v

avoid distortions that are apt to be provoked by fading memories.

This book is not an autobiography of orthodox type. Rather it is a discursive collection of essays sampling the activities and interests that from time to time have dominated my attention throughout a somewhat varied career. In other words it is a medley of autobiographical fragments. Three of the essays are based on lectures that I have given, and these serve to illustrate some of my interests at the time I composed them.

Methodical full-length autobiographies presented in regular sequence from earliest childhood onwards are the privilege of internationally famous men of affairs, a category to which I myself most certainly do not belong. Why, then, do I write of episodes in my life at all? Well, I wrote of them on impulse to begin with, looking back at the excitements and adventures, physical or intellectual, that have given me so much enjoyment during the active days of my career. And then it seemed to me that this short record may be of interest to others, if only by showing that life can indeed be an exciting adventure even when it does not involve record-breaking feats of endurance or exploits of unusual danger. The fact is that we all have a potential capacity for contemplating apparently ordinary events from a slightly unusual angle without in any way distorting them. And if we make use of this capacity we quite commonly discover—with sudden surprise—some element of the extra-ordinary in them.

The frontispiece is reproduced by kind permission of Lady Epstein and Messrs Faber and Faber Limited.

1968   WILFRID LE GROS CLARK

CONTENTS

CHAPTER I

FOREST AND JUNGLE

TODAY, forests and jungles have become scenes of violent strife between man and man. For me this is a melancholy reflection; just those attributes of solitude, remoteness and tangled beauty that in the past have aroused in me feelings pleasantly reposeful and uncoloured by any overtones of disagreeable apprehensions, are now a source of insecurity and hidden dangers in many parts of the world. In contrast, my own reminiscences of journeying uncertainly through little-frequented territories in distant regions are permeated with nostalgic sensations as I call to mind experiences of gentle exploration, and all the suffusions of curiosity and subdued excitement engendered by them.

The last occasion on which I sensed these pleasurable emotions was some years ago in Northern Rhodesia. I was wending my hot and perspiring way through the forested slopes that overlook the southern end of Lake Tanganyika. When I had broken clear of the close packing of scrubby *Brachystegia* woodlands I suddenly came in sight of the lake, a vast, elongated stretch of water that might more appropriately and with well-deserved dignity be called an inland sea rather than a 'lake'. I saw it fading into the vaporous mists of the distance with a cool and placid appearance contrasting rather abruptly with my own sense of effort and fatigue. A few Marabou storks—birds which have claimed as one of their main breeding places the cliffs of the Kalambo Falls nearby—circled lazily in the sky above me and, except for the almost imperceptible rustle and low hum of insects pervading the sun-bedazzled air, all was silent. This was the last of my excursions into such remote territories, and I am filled with regrets that I now have to accept that it was the last. For I think I have enjoyed more than anything else the delights of roving through tropical forests, so frequently have they been a source of physical satisfaction and placid contentment to me. In times of peace it is a recreation providing continuous trains of interest far removed from the petty irritations and trivial anxieties associated with the routine responsibilities of day-to-day life. And sometimes it provides a pleasant titillation of excitement because you are never quite sure from minute to minute what you are likely to come up against next. At each instant of your journey you are surrounded by a circling barrier of trees, but at each step forward the barrier magically opens into a new enclave—and so the process continues incessantly until finally you emerge to find yourself again in more open country. And there is such a remarkable variety in different parts of the tropical world; every geographical type of jungle has its own special and personal qualities that on retrospective reflection tend to isolate themselves in a few salient features from the background of half-conscious recollections. So my memories of the wooded uplands of the central parts of Africa are associated more particularly with acacia trees, aloes and euphorbias, and with buffaloes and baboons and bushbuck. The ubiquitous mangrove forests of equatorial lowlands recall pictures of Nipah palms like gigantic feathers with their glistening pinnate fronds, Rhizophora trees with their aerial roots, mud and mosquitoes, crocodiles and multi-coloured crabs. In the jungles of Malaysia I can visualise the lofty Tapang trees with their buttressing roots spreading out in radiating flanges, orang-utans and argus pheasants, and pitcher plants and pythons. The forested areas of Australia, again, call to mind tree-ferns, blue and scarlet parrots, lyre-birds and opossums, kukkaburras and koala bears.

I suppose it is all this variety, linked with the novelties and

inexpectations of wanderings in jungle and forest, that adds
up to make them so alluring an experience, even though it is an
experience which may sometimes involve physical discomforts,
and frustrating obstructions of many kinds. For one thing, it is
by no means easy to follow little-used tracks through jungle,
and of course even more difficult to cut a pathway where none
existed before. And in equatorial forests there may be pestilen-
tial creatures such as leeches and rather ferocious ants to contend with. Yet, looking back, I would have dearly liked, if
opportunity had offered itself, to sample more different types
of forest and jungle in parts of the earth that I have never
visited. Particularly the forests of the Amazon, because,
indirectly, it was the forests of the Amazon that first gave me
the determination to embark on all the excitements of my own
tropical adventures.

I discovered this one day, many years ago, somewhere near
the middle of Borneo. It was my first expedition up-country
when I had been exploring a small river tributary in a sampan
with two Sea Dyak companions. After an oppressively hot
and humid journey paddling our sampan up the winding
stream and pushing our way through tangles of overhanging
branches, we came to a stretch of forest where I had hoped to
find some of the curious little creatures called tree-shrews—
curious and also very interesting, because these small arboreal
animals have been claimed by some zoologists to represent the
lowest and most primitive grade of that important group of
mammals called the Primates, of which we ourselves, *Homo
sapiens*, are the culminating products of evolutionary development. On landing from our sampan we had laboriously to plod
our way along a jungle track of crude construction made by
the Dyaks at some time or another for their hunting expeditions,
a track composed for the most part of felled tree trunks
(batangs, they call them) that had been manoeuvred into alignment, end to end, a few feet above the swampy undergrowth.

It requires a good deal of care and concentration to negotiate your way along these batangs; like the rest of this particular type of jungle they are soaked in a steamy moisture, and in the course of time become covered with a film of fungoid and algal growth that makes them extremely slippery. The Dyaks with their pliant bare feet can secure a firm enough grip on the rotting surface, but boots, or even soft-soled shoes, are not nearly as efficient for this purpose as the natural corrugations of the skin of the unshod foot. Consequently, with shod feet you tend to slither and slide, and you may even on occasion fall into stagnant pools of water below. Not that this matters much, for in any case your clothes are soon wringing wet with your own perspiration, and from time to time on your journey it may be necessary to wade waist-deep across jungle streams discoloured a rich mahogany brown from the decaying vegetable matter that everywhere floors the forest.

Towards the latter part of the afternoon we came to rising ground where a tract of forest had been cleared some years previously by the local inhabitants for planting rice, and where secondary jungle was beginning to sprout up from an undercoat of rough grass. Here I lay down for a rest, my two Dyak companions squatting beside me quietly smoking their hand-made cigarettes rolled in dried banana leaf. I can very clearly recollect that a troupe of leaf-monkeys were chasing one another with cheerful chuckling cries among the branches of nearby trees, little flights of long-tailed parraqueets every now and again skimmed overhead, and in the distant sky beneath a ceiling of flocculent clouds tinged with a sunset blush a long procession of large fruit-bats, looking very like our own familiar rooks, slowly flapped their way to one of their nocturnal feeding grounds. It was precisely at that moment that I experienced a sudden and intense feeling of contentment and mental ease, interlocked with a sense of quiet exhilaration—as though in this first jungle expedition I had at length achieved the one thing in my life I had always wanted to achieve. This set me on a train of thought; I began lazily to meditate, and to wonder how it was that I ever came to find myself in so delectable a land as Borneo. I could think of several ostensible reasons I had given myself and others for coming there, but now these seemed after all to be only excuses for doing something for which the real motive was very much deeper. Then, in a somewhat dreamy mood I let my mind wander back until, abruptly, I came upon myself as a small boy lying in bed in hospital with scarlet fever; I was reading a boy's story book of the adventures of some explorers in the Amazon forests. I do not remember the title of the book, nor even the details of the adventures. But I do recollect most vividly that the reading of that particular story, combined no doubt with an imagination heightened by my feverish condition, filled me with a tremendous and compelling urge to follow similar adventures for myself if ever I could get the chance to do so. It was with the recollection of this memory that I really came to understand just why I came to be in Borneo—it was the ultimate realization of an emotional urge, an irrational impulse if you like, that had lain latent in my mind since childhood days, and the pretexts I had conjured up for coming to do medical work in this remote tropical country were merely the result of a process of rationalization to provide the opportunity of satisfying this urge.

This vivid personal experience was of considerable interest to me for it revealed to me for the first time that our behaviour and interests and actions, and even our careers in life, are so often ultimately determined by deep-seated impulses of which we may be quite unaware unless we deliberately seek them out by an effort of introspection. Pure reason by itself commonly provides the occasion or opportunity for a course of action, but it does not necessarily engender the inspiration to carry it through to a satisfying conclusion. Pure reason may supply

an ostensible motive, but not the real underlying dictate itself—
it has its importance in guiding and directing a course of action,
but it does not alone generate the drive and momentum to
achieve our ultimate objectives. On the contrary, it is the
irrational impulse that so commonly gives the initial impetus,
and it is the ingrained emotional urge that continues to provide
the real incentive to sustain our energies in working for an end.

It is probably true to say that most boys and girls do not
finally decide on a particular career or profession till quite
late in their growth. This must naturally be so (though most
awkward for parental planning), since it is usually not till
their preliminary education is approaching its terminal stage
that they are in a position to determine for what sort of vocation
they have the necessary talent and in which they are likely to
have an abiding interest. How, indeed, can a youth of fifteen
years be expected to decide finally how he is to spend the next
fifty years of his life? In my own case my career was by a
happy chance of unwitting foresight determined for me at a
very early age. It was while we were quite small children that
my father, a country parson, had quite definite ideas on the
future careers that my two brothers and I should follow. His
plans proved to be mistaken in the case of my brothers, but to
me, the youngest, he had assigned a medical role that eventually
came to realization. This assignment derived from the fact that
both my grandfathers were distinguished in the medical
profession, and my father evidently thought it was due to me
to carry on this family tradition. His own father, Frederick Le
Gros Clark, was a surgeon on the staff of St. Thomas's Hospital;
in his time he was a noted anatomist and in 1874 was President
of the Royal College of Surgeons. I never saw him, for he died
in 1892, three years before I was born. That he had a great
reputation as a surgeon there can be no doubt, otherwise he
would not have achieved the highest distinction to which a
surgeon can aspire. But in his later years he seems to have

become too conservative in his opinions, particularly in regard to the introduction of general anaesthetics for operations. In a book of collected papers published in 1889 he made the following rather surprising reference to this subject. 'Certainly the inhalation of chloroform, or ether, is an almost unmixed boon to the patient. I say almost, because patients seem to suffer more and to experience other inconveniences, when they recover sensibility, than when no chloroform is given. This may be from disappointment on awaking to suffering in the one case, and to a sense of comparative relief when the operation is finished, in the other. Whether anaesthetics are an unmixed advantage to the surgeon I venture to doubt. Formerly the unruliness of a patient could be readily controlled with sufficient assistance; and the operator was, or should have been, too much absorbed with his work, to allow of its being distracted by the patient's inevitable suffering.' These remarks call up a grim picture of operative surgery in pre-anaesthetic days. But my grandfather did go on to say that he had witnessed fatal cases and had himself nearly lost one patient from inhalation, and he also admitted that probably few of his contemporaries would sympathize with his doubts on the subject of general anaesthetics. My mother's father, Edward Clapton, was a physician, also a consultant on the staff of St. Thomas's Hospital. Thus it came about that later on I, too, went to the same hospital to study medicine, and it was during my student days that my smouldering aspirations for tropical adventures were rekindled by reading of the great naturalist explorers of the past such as the account of Darwin's voyage on the *Beagle*, Huxley's travels on the *Rattlesnake*, Bates' wanderings in forests of the Amazon, and Wallace's journeys in the Malaysian Archipelago. This, I thought, was the sort of thing I would like to do, at any rate before I settled down to a permanent career of a more routine nature. However faintly I might copy these paragons of my youth, I would like to catch at least some slight glimmer of the physical and intellectual excitements they themselves experienced. The early career of Alfred Russel Wallace came to have a particular interest for me, partly because his urge to travel in the tropics was in the first instance aroused rather as my own was, though in his case by reading not a boy's adventure story, but a travel book on the Amazon (it was first published in 1847 by an American tourist and entitled *A Voyage up the River Amazon*); partly, also, because in 1854 he visited Malaysia and, while in Sarawak, a country that I later came to know so well myself, wrote a preliminary paper adumbrating his subsequent essay propounding in outline the idea of Natural Selection as the fundamental basis of evolutionary development. It was this essay that precipitated the publication of Darwin's *Origin of Species*, the result of twenty years' enquiry that had led him to formulate precisely the same principle.

When, as a medical student, I came to study human anatomy, I was led to further studies of the relationship of Man with lower animals, in particular his relationship to apes and monkeys that have their natural habitat in equatorial forests and jungles. These interests were for a time interrupted by the First World War, but they sprang up with resumed intensity after my demobilization from the army in 1919. For the ensuing year I was engaged in preparing for the final examination for the Fellowship of the Royal College of Surgeons and, after securing this qualification, in the pursuit of anatomical and anthropological research. But the confines of a laboratory soon became irksome to me, and I experienced a restlessness of mind that at the time I attributed to feelings of disillusionment which the tragedies of war had forced on me. The memories of my work as a medical officer in France, where I had to deal with many terrible mutilations of the wounded during the last phase of fighting before the armistice, were not happy ones. And there were more personal and intimate tragedies that affected me deeply. It was in such a mood of moral perplexity that I was overcome with an intense longing to escape from the artificialities of civilization by losing myself awhile in one of the remoter parts of the world. It was as though, having lost myself in a jungle of conflicting emotions and despondent uncertainties of mind, I felt I might best resolve my perplexities by seeking to disentangle them among the jungles and forests of nature far removed from the conventionalities of my daily life hitherto. At least, this was what I had assumed to be the explanation of my state of mind at the time, until later I came to realize that I was being unconsciously motivated by the subterranean rumblings of an impulse that had its origin far back in my earlier life.

In a vagueness of indecision I consulted an atlas and decided in 1920 to seek a medical post of some kind that would take me either to the Amazon country, or to the Congo, or to Borneo. Any one of these, I thought, would help to satisfy my emotional needs of the moment. Finally, I decided on Borneo, mainly because I knew it to be the home of so many types of animal that interested me—orang-utans, gibbons, a diversity of monkeys, those enigmatical little 'half-monkeys' called tarsiers, and above all, the most primitive creatures akin to the Primates— the tree-shrews. I am sure, also, that my choice was influenced by the little I knew then about the history and people of the island. At any rate, I answered an advertisement for a medical officer on a rubber plantation in British North Borneo (now called Sabah), and having filled up the application form sent to me I was about to return it by post.

It was just on that very day that one of those casual incidents occurred which so often seem almost accidentally to predestine lives and careers of individuals. One of my fellow students who had recently qualified and was about to take up a post in Fiji happened to mention in conversation that a Principal Medical Officer was wanted for Sarawak, the country in

Borneo administered by the third of the 'White Rajahs',
Vyner Brooke. The post, he told me, was not to be advertised
but I could ascertain all the relevant information about it from
the Sarawak Government Office in Millbank. I went straight-
way to the Office and was interviewed by the Rajah's representative there, Mr Willes Johnson, and I had the presumption
to apply for this responsible position, hardly supposing for a
moment that, at the age of twenty-five, my application would
be seriously considered. Yet within a week I was formally
appointed, mainly, I suspect, because of my qualification as a
Fellow of the Royal College of Surgeons. It now seems
strange to me, looking back, that I do not think I had any
foreboding apprehensions of my ability to fulfil the role that I
now found myself cast to play. Strange, because in later life I
have rarely been able to view with equanimity new responsibilities which from time to time I have been led to assume.
My reaction, indeed, was one of great elation. I realized, of
course, that I was ill-equipped in administrative experience to
take medical charge of a country about the size of England and
Wales, but I knew that Sarawak was largely unexplored jungle
and forest. I had no more than a smattering of knowledge of
tropical medicine, but I had four months available to me before
I was due to sail from England and I employed this time in an
intensive course of clinical and laboratory work at the School
of Tropical Medicine in London where facilities were provided
for me by Sir Philip Manson-Bahr.

During this waiting period I also sought all the information
I could about Sarawak by consulting the annual reports of the
Sarawak Government and by reading as many books as I could
obtain having reference to the past history and present condi-
tions of the country and its people, books such as *A History of
Sarawak under its Two White Rajahs* by Baring Gould and
Bamfylde, the two-volume work by Gertrude Jacob on *The
Raja of Sarawak*, Hose and McDougall's *The Pagan Tribes of*

Borneo, A Naturalist in Borneo by Shelford, and many others. So far as the history of Sarawak is concerned, I learnt that a certain James Brooke, who had been severely wounded in the Burmese War in 1825, conceived an impelling desire to return to the Far East to explore the little-known territories of the Malaysian Archipelago. He had become particularly interested in Borneo by reading an account of it by an early traveller, G. W. Earl, published in 1837 under the title of *The Eastern Seas, or Voyages and Adventures in the Indian Archipelago*. The opportunity to satisfy his longings arose when, on the death of his father, he inherited a legacy of £30,000. With this sudden accession of wealth he purchased a schooner of 142 tons, the *Royalist*, assembled a crew, and set sail for Singapore in 1838. From there he paid a visit to Sarawak where he found the country in a state of insurrection and disorder, partly because of the incapacity of the local governor, Makota, who had been appointed by the Sultan of Brunei under whose jurisdiction Sarawak came, and partly because of the misery of the local inhabitants who were continually harried by the piratical incursions of Malays, Sea Dyaks from further up the coast, and Illanuns from the Philippines. Makota found himself incapable of dealing with the situation and sought Brooke's assistance to restore order. This he agreed go do, and as a result of his successful intervention he was offered the sole control of the government of the country with the title of the Rajah of Sarawak. After some delay and, it seems, with some preliminary diffidence, Brooke accepted this offer and his installation in November 1841 met with the ready acquiescence of the whole of the local population with whom he had gained considerable personal prestige. But he had hard times ahead of him in his efforts finally to eradicate piracy, inter-tribal warfare and the ingrained custom of head-hunting, as well as his unremitting struggle to improve the commercial activities of the country in order to reach a favourable trade balance. He

also suffered personal anxieties when in 1853 he almost died
from smallpox and in 1857 narrowly escaped with his life in a
Chinese rebellion that led to the massacre of several Europeans.
Finally he retired to live in the remote village of Burrator on
Dartmoor and died in 1868 after a stroke at the age of sixty-five.
His nephew, later Sir Charles Brooke, succeeded to the title
of the Rajah of Sarawak, and perseveringly continued the
work of the pacification of the country, introducing also many
reforms in its government. After a long reign he died in 1917,
and his son Charles Vyner Brooke succeeded to the Raj; it was
under this third 'White Rajah' that I had been selected as his
Principal Medical Officer. I later came to know Vyner Brooke
well. He had served Sarawak assiduously during his earlier
years as an officer of the government, but it became clear to me
that he was not imbued with the same unwavering drive and
energy that characterized his predecessors; nor, I am sure, did
he have the same zealous interest in his country. He tended to
vacillation in his decisions, evidently the result of some lack of
self-confidence. As a man I found he was genial, friendly, and
generous; too generous, perhaps, for he yielded to favouritism
and came too easily to be influenced by personal advisers who
were not always as wise or scrupulous as they might have been
in their advice.

Having equipped myself with a knowledge of the history
and modern conditions of Sarawak, and having acquainted
myself with the commoner maladies affecting the native population and the treatment required for them, I embarked for this
attractive country on a Blue Funnel Liner, the *Pyrrhus*, which
sailed from Liverpool on 10 October 1920. It would be of
little interest to record all my recollections of the voyage; it was
a common enough experience in those days, and even more so
today. Sarawak is no longer a pleasant little backwater of
civilization to which one journeyed with the anticipatory
excitement of adventuring into the relatively unknown. Now

it is reached within a day or two by air, and lately its jungles and forests have provided commonplace occasions for conducted expeditions by university students and even parties of school-boys. And now, alas, it has been the unhappy scene of political unrest and military activities. In 1920 Sarawak was well off the main traffic lanes of the world, but, even so, I dare say that in the enthusiasm of youth and in my eagerness to seek what to me would certainly be new experiences I tended to invest my journey with a disproportionate sense of glamour. The voyage across the Indian Ocean was to me the most enchanting of my memories. The weather was exquisitely fine, the tang of the tropics in the air became more insistent as a vaguely per-ceptible fragrance wafted across the sea from distant coastlands, and I allowed myself to revel in the newness of sensations that I had not previously experienced. I have sometimes thought that in my wanderings about the world I should have kept a more regular, day-to-day, record of my observations, but I have come to believe I gain more from the novelties of travel by first adopting a passive attitude so that the many impressions are absorbed in their totality, without for a time being dissected into an analysis of separate details. This, it seems to me, is the best way of saturating your mind with the intrinsic atmosphere of new surroundings; it is at a later stage that you should seek to focus attention on their component elements in an attempt to see how they have contributed to the total effect of your experience. But the sum of the parts is never quite equal to the whole, and the latter only comes to full realization by first accepting it as a whole. Thus I allowed myself to fall into a mood of leisurely langour, giving full rein to my senses as we coursed on to Ceylon and thence to Singapore. My most vivid impressions are those of the ocean, its translucent green and caerulean blues in the early morning, and its changes of colour through the cobalt of mid-day to the rich Prussian blue of the late afternoon and then, with the setting of the sun, its transformation into the metallic crinklings of beaten silver. On some nights it was so calm and smooth that single stars in the sky above were reflected as single stars in the sea below, and the motion of the ship was so slight as only to be perceived by the lazy upward and downward swaying of the constellations as I lay watching them from a deck chair.

But my voyage was not one of complete idleness, for during it I made good progress in the study of the Malay language, the *lingua franca* of Borneo. By a fortunate coincidence it happened that at the time of my appointment as Principal Medical Officer the Rajah's brother, by title the Tuan Mudah of Sarawak, was on leave in England and had with him as his personal servant a Malay youth who wanted to return to Sarawak. The Tuan Mudah found it most convenient to get him a passage if he could travel with me as my own personal servant, and on the voyage I made use of him as my instructor in the Malay language. Thus it came about that, by the time I reached Singapore, I had already acquired a working knowledge of colloquial Malay to the extent that I was able to converse in the language in simple terms. I had ten days to spend in Singapore, providing the occasion for purchasing articles of tropical clothing and equipment that I found to be necessary, and then I embarked on a small ship of some 2,000 tons, the *Rajah of Sarawak*, which with its sister ship plied weekly between Singapore and Sarawak. Two days of restful voyaging brought us to Sarawak; the journey was uneventful, and the companionship of fellow travellers returning from leave gave me the opportunity of learning more intimate details of the country for which I was bound. Except for a few small tree-covered islets, the fringing outposts of the little Natuna archipelago, we saw no land until, at dawn, we sighted the coast of Sarawak and slowly passed the wooded limestone headlands of Tanjong Sipang and Tangjong Po to reach the mouth of the Sarawak River at Muara Tebas. From here we crawled slowly up the winding river, following the tortuous bends that here and there, because of their difficult navigation, were placarded with large warning notices such as 'Rocks', 'Hug this shore' and so forth—probably the identical notices that had been standing there since Cuthbert Collingwood referred to them in his book *Rambles of a Naturalist* published in 1868.

It is difficult to find suitable expression for my feelings as I approached Sarawak and penetrated leisurely into its hinterland. The first sight of the coast, bordered with casuarina trees and backed by forested slopes with distant views of mountains still swathed in their early morning mistiness—all this enhanced my excitement, and our sauntering promenade up-river in the silence of the early morning filled me with delight and expectancy. As I looked back over the stern at successive bends of the river the alternate jutting spurs of mangrove forest, fringed with a water-side belt of nipah palms, converged in overlapping sequence like so many folding doors sliding in to shut me off more and more completely from the hurly-burly of the outside world and, in so doing, gave me a pleasing satisfaction that I was about to enter on novel experiences in what was, to me, a different world.

Our final destination was the capital town of Sarawak, Kuching, about twenty miles from the coast along the sinuosities of the river, but considerably closer as measured by a straight line drawn on a map. As we approached it, we began to pass groups of small Malay houses constructed of wood raised on piles, nestling and partly hidden among the surrounding trees. The Malay inhabitants, men, women and children, were taking their morning bath along the river side, and waved happily to us as we glided by. Round the last bend of the river we came in sight of the capital town of Sarawak, Kuching, the buildings glimmering white against a brilliant blue sky, and in the far background the crinkled ridges of the

Matang mountain range at a distance of ten miles or so. Nearing the wharf where we were to disembark, I saw to the right the old fort and the Rajah's residence—the Astana—sited on rising ground, and to the left the town of Kuching fronted by government offices and backed by narrow streets of Chinese shops and markets. Waiting to meet me were the senior Resident Officer, A. B. Ward, the Bishop, Logie Danson (who made it a personal obligation to meet all new-comers to the country), and some of the Chinese members of the medical staff. If I had felt any apprehensions at finding myself a stranger in a strange land, the informality and friendli-ness of my reception put me entirely at my ease. I was taken by the Resident to his house where for a few days I remained the guest of his wife and himself.

During my first few weeks in Sarawak, I learnt much about the country. It reminded me curiously of boyhood stories of remote and long forgotten civilizations hidden in almost inaccessible regions and only rediscovered by enterprising adventurers of the Rider Haggard tradition. Except, of course, that Sarawak was administered by a few of my own country-men, and was visited once a week by a boat bringing passengers, cargo and mail from Singapore. It had its independent govern-ment, with a well-trained police force of Malays and Dyaks and its own little regiment of a few hundred men for use in the occasional isolated disturbances that were still apt to occur up-country. The general status of the country was certainly primitive; there were few roads and these quite local, education-al facilities were poorly developed, and I soon saw many deficiencies in the organization of medical services to which I should need to give rapid attention. But it was a happy country, personal taxation was ridiculously low, and in spite of recent slumps elsewhere in Malaysia these had not appreciably affected the general welfare of the population. At that time the State revenue was somewhat more than two and a half million

(Singapore) dollars, not much, it may seem, to finance the services of a country with an area of 47,000 square miles unless one realized that most of those square miles were occupied by virgin forest, and certainly not adequate for any ambitious schemes of development. But, as I say, it was a happy country, and its contentment and harmony appeared to me all the more remarkable when I considered the extraordinary mixture of the various racial elements of the population, with all their different habits of life, different traditions, different creeds, different languages, and different interests. The record of crime was astonishingly low for so heterogeneous a population, and the sporadic 'incidents' that were occasionally reported near the borders of what was then called Dutch Borneo only served, just because they were sporadic, to emphasize the general peacefulness of the country as a whole. I came quickly to realize that this placid tranquillity was actually based on a deep-rooted and long-standing respect for the Brooke tradition, and also on the administrative efficiency of the civil service. Of course there was a gaol in Kuching for the detention of law-breakers, but it was not called a 'prison'—it was called the 'Sarawak House of Correction' (just as the old penitentiary at Brideswell in London was originally called a House of Correction). Its occupants were allowed an unusual degree of freedom, for they commonly went out during the day to work in private houses or elsewhere, and the normal wages were paid to the Government which passed on a reduced payment to the 'prisoners'. I myself employed in my house a general handy-man (a 'tukang ayer' as we used to call such a worker) who was serving a sentence for manslaughter. He used to arrive on his own soon after six o'clock in the morning, and return to the House of Correction in the afternoon. I remember once, also, interviewing an applicant for work in the Medical Department, and when I asked him what he had recently been doing he replied that he had been working for the Government. It

CPE C

transpired, on further questioning, that he had been serving a sentence for an illegal monetary transaction. Now, I am convinced that he was not trying to deceive me—he was simply expressing the view commonly adopted by inmates of the House of Correction that, having broken one of the laws of the country, he had followed the decision of the court to work (at a reduced pay) for the Government as a just compensation for his infringement of regulations. I employed him in my Department and he always worked satisfactorily.

In my time only about a hundred Europeans comprised the whole of the civil service—Residents, District Officers, Cadets, and those (like myself) who were in charge of special departments. Some were isolated for long periods of time in remote outstations, and others more centrally placed in Kuching or one of the other main towns in the different Divisions of the country. Vyner Brooke, the third Rajah, was not in Sarawak when I arrived; it was his custom to spend rather long intervals of 'leave' in England. But the inspiration and impetus derived from his predecessors, Sir James Brooke and Sir Charles Brooke, still maintained a momentum of administrative zeal and competence that was far from exhausted. In the Rajah's absence, the whole country was under the joint central administration of the Senior Resident, A. B. Ward, and the Treasurer, G. C. Gillan. My regard for the administrative officers in general increased as I came to know them more intimately. On first acquaintance they might give an impression of a leisureliness of habit that could be mistaken for a languorous mentality associated with a too easy attitude towards their responsibilities. But this was far from being the case. Behind their quiet and unassuming demeanour, the Residents and District Officers, with very few exceptions, concealed an earnestness and resoluteness of purpose in their work. I am glad to pay this tribute to my Sarawak colleagues of almost half a century ago, for it occasionally happened that some visitors who had made but a brief stay in the country, and thus gained no real insight into the complexities of its administration or the sort of problems that the latter involved, threw quite unjust aspersions on the administrative personnel of the time. I think particularly of a book written by a man of Scandinavian extraction who was, during my Sarawak days, a temporarily appointed curator of the Kuching Museum. I later read his book in a French translation, with the somewhat magniloquent title *Borneo. L'Isle des Chasseurs de Têtes*. The author, by his rather abrupt mannerisms and his petty grumblings about his appointment, did not achieve the popularity with his fellows that he might have done. Perhaps he realized this and for that reason was led to make scurrilous attacks on government officials, accusing them among other things of gross inefficiency and lassitude. The same author wrote another book of a popular nature on the natural history of Sarawak, published in an English edition and entitled *Forest Life & Adventures in the Malay Archipelago*; in the preface he made the extravagant remark, 'Many a time death stared me in the face.' I suppose, if I wished to impress readers with imaginary dangers, I could by a little amplification, not too scrupulously presented, record similar excitements in my own experience. For example, I once encountered a king cobra in the porch of my house; on a few occasions I met with scorpions in my bathroom; in search of a rare type of monkey I once waded through a muddy mangrove swamp inhabited by crocodiles; on a visit to a small island off the coast of Borneo I seized the opportunity for a sea bathe, which I was afterwards told was a silly thing to do because that particular island is a well-known resort for turtle breeding and the sea is frequented by sharks on the look-out for newly-hatched turtles; and one day on a journey through jungle a large python crossed my pathway. But I am not able truthfully to record that on any of these occasions did death stare me in the face. The cobra was lying coiled up in a quiet reverie and was easily despatched with a blow of a heavy stick. Scorpions are readily avoidable with a little care. I did not see any crocodiles in that mangrove swamp (though I saw the tracks of one). I enjoyed a most refreshing bathe off my turtle island in water so transparently clear that, swimming below the surface, I marvelled at the chromatic variegations of corals and sea anemones and their attendant shoals of tropical fish, but I encountered no sharks. And the python glided so quickly out of my way that it seemed far more frightened of me than I was likely to be of it.

I recollect only one occasion when I was apprehensive during my years in Sarawak, and in retrospect that now appears only amusing. I had travelled up-country and was walking over a hilly district intersected with deep ravines of mountain streams. I came to a gorge-like valley that had to be crossed by a long and narrow tree-trunk felled across it from one side to the other. I had not the courage on my outward journey to walk erect over this primitive bridge (which of course had no supporting rails) and so I straddled across it in a sitting position. On my return I was about to assume the same undignified method of transit when a group of Dyaks appeared on the other side and politely waited for me to cross over first. A sense of self-pride impelled me to overcome my fears, and with considerable trepidation I walked upright along the uneven and slippery surface, striving to avoid giddy side-glances at the rushing and swirling river torrent some hundred feet below. Fortunately I accomplished this bit of space travel successfully, but with a profound feeling of relief and a silent prayer of thanksgiving on reaching the other side.

As a preparation for my medical and administrative work, on my arrival in Sarawak I made a tour of inspection of hospitals and dispensaries in Kuching and elsewhere, including some of the further outstations, making the acquaintance of all the members of my medical staff, and familiarizing myself with the organization of the medical services of the country as a whole. I soon came to realize that my medical experiences were to be very varied indeed, but I will defer reference to them here for they follow in better sequence to my brief narrative of clinical work at St. Thomas's Hospital and in the army during the war. When I returned to Kuching from my tour I moved into the house that had been allocated to me, a house of bungalow type placed beyond the outskirts of the town in a somewhat isolated position. It had an inviting garden which was a pattern in miniature of the tropical jungle of Malaysia, but it was a tidy jungle for my Malay gardener kept the grassy slopes smooth with his skilful scythe-work and also tended the few beds of cannas and hibiscus that sprinkled small patches of reds and yellows bringing out in stronger contrast the all-pervading greens. Scattered here and there were clusters of graceful nibong palms and compact groups of the more delicate areca-nut palm. In one corner a thicket of bamboos stood alongside irregular straddles of pineapple plants and banana trees. Bordering the entrance to the garden was a grove of coconut palms, some grown quite tall and others in their infancy with fronds spraying fountain-wise straight from the ground. Near the house (as a reminder of one of the main industries of Malaysia) stood a loose screen of rubber trees. And, dominating the scene as viewed from my verandah, was a splendid specimen of one of the larger forest trees, a shorea, the solitary relic of the primary forest that at one time must have been cleared to provide, unwittingly, a space for me to live in.

I learnt very early in my Sarawak days that, in order to keep in vigorous health in a humid equatorial climate, consistent and energetic physical exercise is essential. There were plenty of facilities for this—rides on my pony 'Kluang' between six and seven o'clock in the morning along grass tracks among the Malay kampongs, hard sets of tennis in the evening, badminton, and other games. But I derived my greatest pleasure from excursions into surrounding tracts of jungle. About two miles from Kuching is a small tree-covered hill, Bukit Siul, and leading to it was a primitive and much overgrown jungle path, hardly altered, I suspect, since it was described by the Italian botanist Beccari over a hundred years ago in his travel book *Wanderings in the Great Forests of Borneo*. I used to make this journey from time to time, starting out just before full daylight and reaching the summit of the hill to watch the sun rising over the forest around me and bringing to a glow the buildings of Kuching below. This excursion took its way along ill-defined tracks partly obscured by obstacles of interwoven roots and creepers, and in some places where the ground was swampy it could only be accomplished by way of elevated batang 'viaducts' constructed from tree trunks. It traversed what is called secondary jungle, that is to say, the tangled up-growth of vegetation that rapidly springs from the soil where primary jungle had been cleared at some previous time. Here, multitudes of trees and shrubs and climbing plants seem to be engaged in a wild scramble to establish themselves in fierce competition with each other. It is on such journeys that the Malay parang is an indispensable implement, for you have literally to hack your way step by step.

Primary jungle, or more dramatically, primaeval forest, was also quite near Kuching, across the river from my house and towards the Matang range. To wander through this tract of country was less arduous than through secondary jungle because the undergrowth is much less dense, and in places altogether absent. Primaeval forest represents the terminal phase in the struggle for existence between competing trees; by now those which have won in the rivalry have stretched up to the skies to reach a height of two hundred feet or more above the ground, their massed foliage at the top supported by serried pillars of enormous trunks. But the latter are not completely naked, for many are entwined with climbing creepers that make use of them as ladders to struggle their own way up to the sunlight. Others are festooned with hanging lianas, or here and there are bedecked with orchids of great variety. The forest is carpeted with a floor of soft humus and leaf mould, and, although not dark, by contrast with the burning glare of daylight outside it appears on first entering it to be dim and gloomy. But this is no more than a first impression, for here and there the sun strikes through where a tree has at one time crashed in a storm, bringing down with it (as it commonly does) its immediate neighbours that may be entangled in the same creepers. In these occasional glades lace-winged butterflies flap so gently and leisurely as to give a slow-motion effect, but except for these and other insects, as well as the ubiquitous leeches, the primary forest seems by day to be almost lifeless. In the middle of the day, indeed, it is pervaded with a rather eerie silence which, according to their accounts, has led travellers to feel they are all the time being watched by unseen eyes. The silence, and the apparent lack of animal life, is due to several factors. Most of the life of primary forest is being actively pursued, especially during the early morning and the cool of the evening, in the canopy of the tree tops; here is the attic world of the forest birds, of squirrels and tree-shrews, of bands of monkeys or families of gibbons and, in certain restricted parts of Sarawak, of the retiring and unsociable orang-utan. Down below, such creatures as may inhabit the lower levels of the forest, or descend in the heat of the day to the protective shadiness beneath the foilage, can easily elude the observer by hiding among the enveloping palisades of tree trunks so that they are rarely seen. The softness of the forest floor, also, dulls the sound of footsteps like a rich plush carpet, and sounds in the near distance tend to be absorbed and muffled by the continuous roof of foliage above. But not all is quiet. The rushing noise of a hornbill far above can be heard from time to time, while in the early part of the morning or in the late afternoon an argus pheasant, one of the most beautiful of forest birds, may betray its presence somewhere near by its shrill cry, or now and again the cheerful, bubbling chorus of gibbons echoes among the trees.

In my wanderings through the forests of Borneo, whether in mangrove swamps, in lowland areas of primary and secondary jungle, or over wooded hills and mountains, I wished I had acquired a botanical knowledge that would have enabled me to identify the various trees, creepers, epiphytes, and so forth, among which I journeyed. The giant trees of the primary forest at first sight look much alike to the unsophisticated eye, but this is mainly because their distinguishing foliage is far above, while their trunks are not so conspicuously different. Many of them have this in common, that the base of the trunk sends out great flanges that serve as buttresses to give the support needed where the soil or the limited surrounding space does not permit of deep and widely spreading roots. I learnt to recognize the shorea tree and other dipterocarps that provide commercial timber, the jelutong tree that yields uncultivated rubber, the ironwood or bilian tree (a wood so dense that it sinks in water and is impervious even to the depredations of the destructive white ant), pandanus palms sheltering unobtrusively like midgets in the shade of the titans surrounding them, the climbing rattan palm with its treacherous spiky thorns, and several kinds of low-lying ferns. I was surprised, also, to find such an astonishing variety of fig trees of so many contrasting types. Some grow as small bushes; others spring up mightily and align themselves with other giants of the forest. Still others grow down from above; their seeds having been deposited by birds in the forked branches of tall trees, they germinate there and send down great aerial roots that seek and eventually find the ground. I have good reason to remember these aerial roots, for on one occasion during an expedition with some Kayan natives through the forests in

northern Sarawak, loss of body water from the heat-induced
perspiration soon gave me an overwhelming thirst. But this
was easily quenched, for one of my Kayan companions cut out
a two-foot section of a root and told me to hold it up with the
lower end to my mouth. There trickled out a flow of cool pure
water, such as might come from a fresh mountain spring. But I
think the most exquisitely refreshing drink to quench one's
thirst was provided by the occasional coconut trees that we
met in the neighbourhood of native dwellings in the jungle; the
milk from coconuts imported into Europe is insipid or sickly
sweet, bearing no comparison with the milk of nuts cut down
anew from trees growing on the spot. There is no need to
carry a supply of water on a jungle expedition for, apart from
aerial roots and coconuts, there is always abundant water to be
obtained from a variety of sources—from rain collected in the
fronds of palms, or from springs and small streams in hilly
districts.

To see the panorama of jungle and forest in Borneo in
all its magnificent aspect, it should be viewed from a height.
About one thousand feet up the eastern flank of the Matang
range was a small bungalow, and here I sought an occasional
rest of a few days when I could spare the time from my
medical work. Looking down over the flat country below I
could see the canopy of primary forest stretching for miles
towards the sea, the foliage of the tops of individual trees making
in the distance an almost continuous surface of rumpled, moss-
like corrugations, here and there interrupted by smoother
islands of a lighter green that marked patches of secondary
jungle. In the distance some tree-covered hills take on a
bluish tinge and beyond them is a misty indication of the
coastal plain and the sea. Towards the evening the oblique rays
striking from the setting sun throw the corrugations of the
canopy into sharper relief, and as the sun submerges below the
horizon—changing the day to night with an abruptness that

contrasts with the delaying twilight of higher latitudes—the forest seems suddenly to come alive with the activities of little creatures whose existence is unsuspected during the day. These are the cicadas, described in the formal language of an encyclopaedia as 'insects of the homopterous division of the Hemiptera'. They vary greatly in size, but they have this in common—the males are equipped on the side of the abdomen with a drumlike membrane that can be made to vibrate at a high frequency by muscular action, producing a noise which in some cases may be amplified by a sort of miniature sounding-board. The intensity of the sound is quite astonishing in relation to the size of the insect and it may be audible over a distance of a quarter of a mile or more. There are many different species of cicada, each of them making a characteristic noise that is assumed to act as a sexual stimulus to the female. These stridulating love-calls begin to make themselves heard at the onset of darkness, the first of them almost precisely as the sun sets, and because near the equator this occurs at about six o'clock the creature responsible for it is called by the Malays the 'kriang pukul anam', that is, the 'six o'clock cicada'. Many travellers in Malaya and Borneo have made reference to this, and several of them (perhaps in repetition from reading descriptions of previous writers) have likened the noise to a high-pitched braying of a donkey. But to my mind it is not so discordantly harsh as that; it is more like the sound of blowing in and out the treble notes of a mouth-organ. Other kinds of cicada soon come also into play; one sounds rather like a distant saw-mill, another like the twittering of a grass-hopper, one gives off a low vibrating hum, and another imitates a referee's whistle blown every now and again in one or two short blasts as if a football match were in progress somewhere close by. One particular cicada attracted my attention on my Matang nights because it gave out a series of twangs resembling the preliminary tuning up for a concert of string instruments. This was to me a very apt simile, for when all the cicadas got going together they seemed in combination to form an orchestral fantasia, and in low-lying jungle this often has an intermittent bass accompaniment of croaking frogs.

To newcomers in Borneo the nightly chorus of cicadas may at first be disturbing to the ear, giving the impression of a dissonant cacophony not very conducive to sleep. But it later resolves itself into what it really is—the natural symphony of the nocturnal forest, a symphony that is not without its own intrinsic harmony. After a time the ear becomes numbed to the sounds of the jungle and they cease to be consciously perceived unless the chorus suddenly stops for a few moments, as it sometimes does, and then the abrupt stillness by its very contrast awakens an attitude of tense alertness. Involuntarily you strain to listen; in fact, the whole jungle seems to be straining to listen. What is it, I have wondered, that determines these intervals of silence among such multitudes of different creatures? Presumably a call uttered by some bird or beast is taken as an alarm signal for a momentary pause, but the pause never lasts long, and the concert is renewed as suddenly as it ceased.

The tropical forest at night is a source of wonderment and awe, but in the morning it attains to a sublimity of quiet beauty. When the sun begins slowly to lift itself up from the horizon in the creation of another dawn, the canopy of the forest over the plains is no longer visible from the mountain heights; it is draped in an unbroken sheet of silvery mist that stretches as far as the eye can see. Then, with the growing warmth of the sun, the mist is drawn upwards into streaming wreaths of white vapour, so that the whole vastness of the forest looks afire. But all this rapidly dissipates into slender wisps of haze, or here and there congeals into more compact clouds floating slowly away and baring the tree-tops into full visibility. If there are scattered hills and valleys in the landscape their contours become outlined and sculptured by the drifting clouds that, cleaving into valleys and hollows, bring to notice irregularities of contour not previously observed. Finally, the low-lying clouds vanish altogether, and the irregularities merge once more into a general flatness smoothed out by the more vertical rays of sunlight. The restful pleasure of my early mornings on Matang was enhanced by the circumstance that immediately behind the bungalow was a slender waterfall cascading down a rocky face into a pool below, and here I was able to enjoy a natural shower-bath of spray that felt so icy cold as to make me catch my breath and instil an invigorating sense of well-being.

I wish my official duties had permitted me to explore forest regions still further afield in Borneo, though I had occasion sometimes to do so when visiting isolated native communities round some of the more remote outstations for medical inspection and treatment. But I never had the opportunity of penetrating very far into the moss forest of the higher mountains. I had but a glimpse of their characteristic vegetation, shrouded in almost continuous mist, when I climbed about 3,000 feet up one mountain. But the fully developed moss forest begins at about the 3,500-foot level. Here the trees become stunted and gnarled into distortions reminiscent of some of Arthur Rackham's drawings of haunted woods. Their branches are draped with dripping clumps of moss, and it is particularly here that orchids abound, as well as a great diversity of insectivorous pitcher plants of curious shape that in some species are blotched with colours of unexpected brilliance. It has been well said that the pitcher plant is one of the most distinctive features of the Bornean forest, and its elaborate mechanism for trapping insects and digesting them with some sort of proteolytic enzyme adds a bizarre touch to its exquisitely proportioned beauty.

An excursion into equatorial jungle may sometimes be an

arduous experience, a matter of blood, sweat and toil. Toil because of the difficulties of circumventing tangled pathways and clambering over slippery tree roots; sweat, because of the incessant and profuse perspiration evoked by the humid heat; and blood, because of the lively activity of mosquitoes and leeches. Biting ants also make themselves a nuisance in the forest, and on one occasion my companions and I found our path obstructed by a closely packed and uninterrupted column of ants on a migratory march, looking like an interminable brown serpent adorned with a skin of shimmering scales. We had to light a fire to deflect them into another direction. But all these hazards of jungle wanderings seem relatively trivial by comparison with the excitement of the novelties they presented to me.

Now I would not have it supposed from what I have said in this chapter that I have any wish to pose as the sort of 'intrepid explorer' often associated with travel stories of fact and fiction. I am not that sort of person at all. My wanderings in the forests of Borneo were no more than interludes in a very busy life of medical work, even though this work often provided the opportunity for such interludes because it called for occasional journeys into the more remote interior of the country. It might be thought, also, from these references to my Sarawak days that my experience of the country was much more extensive and intimate than it really was. After all, I only spent three years in Borneo, but these were the formative years of my career, its first chapter so to speak, and their effects have dominated much of my attitude to life ever since. Cogitating on the driving power of the instinctive impulse for exploration, I later came to realize how much I owed to my sporadic adventures in tropical forests. At the time, also, I found that the alertness of mind necessary to cope with immediate eventualities in jungle journeys by a kind of compensatory mechanism came to be balanced by a relaxation of attention on subjective anxieties and worries, and so reduced them to the trivialities they turned out to be.

My mind is filled with so many glad memories of my excursions into the interior of Borneo interwoven with my medical duties and, indeed, often occasioned by these duties— journeys along the winding rivers and at sea up and down the coast; staying in the 'long-houses' of Dyaks, watching their dancing, and sleeping under a festoon of dried human heads hanging from the roof (relics of their head-hunting days); the excitements of tuba fishing; learning to catch fresh-water prawns by casting the jala-jala net; exploring labyrinthine caves filled with swiftlets and their edible bird-nests and with multitudinous bats; my early rides at daybreak enjoying the fresh coolness of the morning air; and moonlight bathing off coastal shores. But of all my memories of Sarawak my garden stands out most clearly because, I suppose, I used to contemplate this so regularly in the evening. I see myself sitting on my verandah at night, after a hard day's work, and I see my garden under a calm and starry sky with the southern constellations scintillating in brilliant sparkles against a background of darkest violet. And when the moon is full it floodlights the lofty shorea tree to make it stand out against the dim outlines of bamboos and coconut trees below. The fronds of the palm trees glisten, silver-edged by the moon, and a faint breeze gives a delicious sense of coolness after the sweltering heat of a tropical day. And, as background music to this reposeful diorama, there are the strains of my own private cicada orchestra, accompanied by the erratic rhythm in a lower key of the croakings of frogs.

*   *   *   *   *   *

I have written about Sarawak as I knew it, Sarawak as it was almost fifty years ago. If in those days it was still a primitive and relatively undeveloped country, it was a happy country so far as happiness may be expressed in terms of the contentment of the people under a paternal and efficient administration in which they had full confidence, and the mutual harmony that bound together communities made up of such a diversity of racial elements with all the complexities of their contrasting modes of life. But the days of Brooke rule are now over, and they ended with tragic abruptness. The centenary of Sir James Brooke's accession to the Raj was celebrated in September 1941, and on the following Christmas Day the Japanese occupied Kuching after over-running much of the rest of the country. The third Rajah, Sir Vyner Brooke, had gone on one of his long 'leaves' not long before the invasion, so that, as Steven Runciman remarks in his history of Sarawak *The White Rajahs*, 'At this miserable crisis of her history there was no Brooke in Sarawak'. The country had been left in the charge of the Chief Secretary. This is no occasion for recounting the horrors and atrocities of the Japanese occupation of Sarawak. The miseries and hardships suffered by those interned in the prison camps near Kuching have been made clear by Agnes Keith in her book *Three came home*, and by Michael O'Connor in *The more fool I*. The cruelties inflicted by the Japanese on their prisoners were systematic and premeditated. The terrible massacre of men, women and children who had sought refuge in the small out-station of Long Nawang in the interior of the country, the sadistic reprisals against the local inhabitants of some of the towns who did not conform strictly to all the orders of the invaders, the wanton and summary execution of innocent civilians—none of these can be mentioned without most disturbing emotions.

The final tragedy of Sarawak prisoners took place in North Borneo. In 1944, the Japanese authorities in Kuching accused the Chief Secretary and four others of smuggling into the prison camp a Chinese newspaper. Although the accusation was unfounded, all of them were 'tried' by court-martial under the direction of the Japanese secret police, the Kempitai, and they were transferred to Jesselton to serve hard sentences of several years. Unfortunately, units of the Australian army landed in North Borneo in 1945 before the war in the Far East was terminated by atom bombs, and the Japanese did what they certainly intended to do with all their prisoners in the event of a land attack—they killed them. Later a message was found crudely carved on a tree trunk in their jungle prison by the Chief Secretary; it read 'I, with the Consul General, Dr Stookes, MacDonald and Webber, have been taken to Keningau. Allied bombers now come every day and I feel that landings are about to take place. But my life is soon to be taken and, when victory comes, only my words written here will remain.' After the surrender of the Japanese it was revealed at the trial of those responsible for committing this atrocity on civilian prisoners that a friendly native had built a shelter in an almost inaccessible part of the jungle, stocked it with food, and tried to persuade the five men to escape to it. But, although they had an opportunity to do so while hiding in local jungle during air raids, they consistently refused this opportunity because they knew well enough that, if they did, the local inhabitants would be subjected to terrible reprisals. Of course, this is only one instance of agonizing sufferings of prisoners in the Far East ending in their death. But it was a particularly poignant tragedy for me, for the Chief Secretary was my brother, Cyril. He had joined the Sarawak Civil Service in 1925, two years after my return to England, and gained rapid promotion by his administrative ability until he came to occupy the most senior position in the Sarawak Government under the Rajah. As Chief Secretary he had initiated a number of important administrative reforms leading to a more democratic form of government. A fine memorial, dedicated to him and to all those of all races who lost their lives in the cause of Sarawak, has now been erected in Kuching, and another memorial to him and his four comrades has also been placed at Keningau where they were killed on the very eve of liberation.

How long, one wonders, will these memorials remain? Recent history has shown that too often memorials to distinguished administrators and others who have been concerned for the prosperity and happiness of the people under their care have been removed and destroyed under the direction of new administrations. And, as I write, the very existence of Sarawak as we have known it in the past has been threatened from without.

CHAPTER 2

ON KEEPING BODY AND SOUL TOGETHER

THE phrase 'keeping body and soul together' is usually taken to refer to the boundary between life and death. In fact, it can be given a far wider connotation, for the mildest of illnesses leads to a slight disjunction between the two, in the sense that the mind and body for the time being are not in complete harmony with one another. A severe cold in the nose, for example, effects a trifling, but nonetheless real, modification in our mental attitude towards the circumstances of our life, and tends for a time to disrupt the evenness of our temperament. In serious illnesses the breach between mind and body may be more obtrusive, but only in fatal terminations does the detachment become complete. Thus it may be said that the task of the physician has always the aim of maintaining or restoring the complete equilibrium between the two that is characteristic of the normal healthy individual.

It surprises me to read lectures expounded from time to time by medical pundits appearing to call in question the concepts of diseases as distinct entities and stressing the self-evident fact that attention should be focussed on the reactions of individual patients to disordered functions and not only on the specificity of the agent of the disease. It surprises me because such admonitions seem to be unnecessary. When I was a medical student it was continually impressed on us that every patient should be considered as an individual with a personality of his own, and that in dealing with them we were dealing with human beings whose attitudes of mind in the course of their illness always need careful and sympathetic consideration. But even if this had not been impressed on us by our clinical teachers, we could not fail to realize it ourselves in the course of our daily work in the wards. The fact is that as dressers in the surgical wards or clinical clerks in the medical wards, and later on as house surgeons or house physicians, we were in far more intimate contact with our patients than some of the visiting consultants. For whereas we would see the patients under our care every day, or several times during each day and night, and in conversation with them learn all their personal anxieties and hopes and fears, the consultant might visit them but briefly only once or twice a week. Similarly, the general practitioner cannot help but familiarize himself with each of his patients as *individuals*, and not merely as so many outward manifestations of 'diseases' to be neatly catalogued and labelled according to the categories listed in text-books. I suspect, indeed, that the lectures to which I have referred are mainly the expositions of those specialists, or clinical research workers in laboratories, who having lost contact with the individualities of patients are prone to overlook them—the lectures are unconsciously aimed at correcting their own tendencies to regard diseases as pure abstractions and not really to draw the attention of the general practitioner to the obvious. But I would also claim that the various diseases that affect mankind are indeed entities, in so far as they are for the most part determined by some specific agent, known or as yet unknown, whether this agent is a pathogenic micro-organism, or the result of a biochemical defect in metabolism, or a malignant growth of one particular type or another. Since human beings are very like one another anatomically, physiologically and biochemically, they commonly react to these agents of disease very similarly. But all human beings are not *exactly* alike—particularly in mentality and temperament, and to this extent, of course, their reactions are not perfectly duplicated as between one individual and another. All this is surely well-known, yet even when individual variations are taken into account the nature of most illnesses can be recognized by the physical signs and symptoms to which they give rise. In this sense, evidently, diseases are entities in the usually accepted sense of the term. Thomas Sydenham, no doubt one of the most pre-eminent among the early physicians of the seventeenth century, wrote that 'although there are varieties in the symptoms of disease, yet Nature acts in so orderly a manner that the same disease appears with like symptoms in different persons'. Incidentally, Sydenham's portrait hangs in my own College at Oxford, Hertford College, and he was one of the most distinguished worthies of his time.

Of course the subjective reaction of each individual to a physical illness varies, the more so the graver the disorder. There are those who yield too easily to melancholy and despair; they either succumb rapidly or can only be persuaded to recover by continual exhortation and encouragement. It is in such cases that the personality of the physician is of primary importance in accelerating a cure. There are also those who face disabilities or incurable complaints with a fortitude and cheerfulness that always fills me with the deepest admiration for the potential courage and tenacity of the human mind in the face of extremes of adversity. The term 'psychosomatic' has now come to find a permanent place in medical diction. It may perhaps be sometimes too easily applied to disorders whose physical basis is obscure—a confession of ignorance on the part of the diagnostician. But it has rightly been said that all illnesses are psychosomatic to the extent that the somatic or bodily symptoms can be to a greater or lesser extent modified by the mental attitude of the patient towards them. All these principles that should determine right relations between doctor and patient were first instilled into me during my course of medical training as a student at St. Thomas's Hospital.

I left Blundell's School at an early age, for I had been fortunate enough to pass the London Matriculation examination at the age of sixteen. It was in 1912, therefore, that I entered London University as a medical student at St. Thomas's Hospital where both my grandfathers had established a fine family tradition by their distinguished careers on the consultant staff many years previously. The change from school to university can have a very enlightening effect on a receptive mind, and as my own mind was filled with an eagerness and excitement for learning it was certainly receptive. At school we acquire knowledge usually at second or third hand, for it is uncommon for our teachers to be outstanding authorities on the subjects that they teach (though some are). In a university, there is greater opportunity to come into direct contact with men and women who are themselves engaged in the exciting task of intellectual discovery in the very subjects that they teach, for most are also occupied in original research. Thus we actually see new discoveries being made around us at the very time we are discovering new knowledge for ourselves—it is as though we almost become active participants (instead of distant lookers-on) in the task of assembling new facts and the development of new ideas. All this contributes to a sense of intellectual adventure that stirs and inspires the imagination.

At St. Thomas's Hospital Medical School our lecturer on physics was Mr Brinkworth, who delivered his lectures with a remarkable lucidity and contrived the most ingenious practical exercises for us to carry out. He even brought us up to the stage where we could, by our own efforts of reasoning, calculate the velocity of a hydrogen atom—no mean feat in a course of instruction lasting only one year. Dr Le Sueur and Dr Haas took us in organic and inorganic chemistry; both were recognized authorities in these subjects and not only introduced us to their fundamentals but carried us forwards to a consideration of chemical problems currently under discussion. The lecturer in biology, the late Dr Ruggles Gates, was a distinguished scientist, but distinguished in a rather narrow field. He was a dreary lecturer and tended to focus his attention too exclusively on his own research interests to the detriment of many other aspects of biology which to some of us seemed more important. He used to get unmercifully ragged because of his attempts to discipline us as though we were still schoolboys. On one occasion he locked the door of the practical classroom in order to prevent us from leaving before time was up. A silly thing to do, for next day in the late afternoon he found himself locked in his own laboratory, and it was some time before he managed to draw attention to his predicament.

After successfully circumventing the examinations in the preliminary subjects of chemistry, physics and biology, I passed on to the preclinical sciences, anatomy and physiology. The professor of anatomy was F. G. Parsons, a man who was almost a caricature of the professor of fiction because of his absent-mindedness. He was by no means a good lecturer, but he was unusually skilful in blackboard artistry, and he made up for his hesitant, rambling, and often disconnected sentences by the clarity of his very engaging diagrams. Indeed, he would often spend hours before one of his lectures preparing these illustrations with coloured chalks, and giving them a perspective by bringing out the high-lights in white chalk after the manner of the pavement artists of that time. Since his own interests were primarily in the field of comparative anatomy and evolutionary morphology, subjects that particularly interested me as a student, I derived a considerable stimulus from the instruction we received from him, even though his disquisitions often bore little relation to the needs of the medical curriculum. It interested me to discover that, on entering the dissecting-room for the first time and seeing a number of human corpses laid out on tables in preparation for the term's work, I experienced no emotional qualms of any kind, in spite of the fact that I had never before seen a recently dead body. But they looked very much like the mummies displayed in archaeological museums, and I accepted them as a matter of course as 'specimens' for dissection, just as I had accepted in our biological curriculum the preserved specimens of dog-fish, frog and rabbit for dissection. The actual process of dissection was an adventure of exploration in itself— removing the skin to display superficial nerves, lymphatics and blood vessels, exposing the muscles one by one and considering by reference to their position and attachments how they are used during life, tracing out arteries and veins and following all their main branches and tributaries, and examining with one's own eyes the vital organs of circulation, digestion, respiration and reproduction that not so long previously had been full of action. It was like exploring a new geographical territory, surveying and charting the organs of the body with the detail necessary for constructing a mental atlas that would later enable one to visualize, as an imaginary transparency, the internal topography of patients whose ailments required a diagnosis.

John Mellanby was the professor of physiology, shy and diffident in manner but a very effective lecturer; he obviously prepared his lectures with great care, and introduced a clear perspective into a subject where it was easy to lose one's way for a time in the diffuseness of some of the formal text-books then available to us. I found the practical classes in physiology somewhat less satisfying than those in anatomy, mainly because at that time we were supplied with apparatus of rather poor construction so that we might have to spend a good deal of frustrating time getting the apparatus to work before we could achieve any experimental results. We also wasted a great deal of time over practical histology, for we had to stain and mount all our own microscopical sections individually, and with our inexperience we finished up with preparations that were often technically poor or indifferent. The classes in

chemical physiology (now called biochemistry) were more
stimulating, though in my days very limited in scope.

After the preclinical phase of the medical curriculum, on to
clinical work—'walking the wards' as it used to be termed. It
is but natural that to many medical students the transition from
preclinical to clinical studies comes as a great relief, for the
former sometimes appear to them as so much drudgery to be
endured, and to be finalized by searching examinations, before
starting on what is the real objective of their life's work—the
care and treatment of human patients. In my own case it was
not quite so, for I had enjoyed my preclinical studies in the
basic sciences; they certainly involved work that was hard and,
at times, wearying, for in those days we had to learn and
memorize factual details in far greater quantity than the
modern medical student is usually required to do. To me, one
of the major attractions of the clinical course lay in the opportunity it provided for the exercise of intellectual skill and
ingenuity in diagnosis. And the excitement of these intellectual
exercises was accentuated by a sense of urgency because the
arrival as soon as possible at a correct diagnosis was so clearly a
matter of the utmost importance to the suffering patient. We
were dealing with fellow beings, anxious and uncertain about
themselves or about those closely bound up with them in love
and affection, and if their ailments presented a riddle to be
solved the solution was to be sought with all speed so as to
apply the appropriate remedy most likely to effect a cure if this
should be feasible, or at any rate to give some measure of
relief.

So we applied ourselves to learning the whole elaborate
technique of diagnosis, recording the medical history of the
patient and his family, enquiring into the details of all the
symptoms that he had observed for himself, and by our own
examination eliciting the 'physical signs' that might indicate
the nature of the disorder. This examination depended, in

regular order, on inspection, palpation, percussion and auscultation. By inspection we trained our powers of visual observation and discovered that the experienced eye may be able from time to time to diagnose with certainty many types of bodily disorder, even without the necessity for further examination. Palpation cultivated our sense of touch so that we came to recognize a slight tell-tale rigidity where the tissues should normally be soft and pliable, a slight resistance where there should be resilience, a slight irregularity of contour or size of underlying organs palpable from the surface. Percussion, or tapping with the finger, by detecting abnormalities of hollowness or solidity, gave us clues to cavities that ought not to exist, to the presence of pathological fluids in or around hollow viscera, or to the enlargement or displacement of solid organs. This technique of percussion was simple in principle, but it only yielded relevant information after prolonged practice. It used to remind me of the stone-mason, Durdles, in Dickens' unfinished novel *The Mystery of Edwin Drood*; by tapping with his hammer on a stone wall, Durdles claimed that he could detect solid underneath, or hollow, or even solid in hollow and yet again hollow in solid. Of course, by digital percussion it is not possible to analyse differences in the percussion 'note' with such precision as this, but I was surprised to find what information about the deeper tissues of the body could be obtained by this method. Then, by auscultation with a stethoscope, one learnt to distinguish the warning murmurings of a distressed heart, the significance of a great variety of abnormal sounds in infected lungs, the pulsating swish of a deep-seated aneurysm, and so forth. By collating the details of the medical history, the patient's symptoms, and the various physical signs that we discovered by our own examination, it was usually possible to fit them into a reasonably neat jigsaw pattern that revealed the real nature of the malady. But in many cases we had to supplement all this information, before we could arrive at a sure diagnosis, by special tests of a bacteriological nature, by radiography, chemical analysis of body fluids, microscopical examination of the blood, and other technical procedures.

As medical students with the status of clinical clerks or surgical dressers we were constantly and carefully supervised by a whole hierarchy of highly qualified and experienced clinicians; beyond the house physicians and house surgeons there were the Resident Assistant Physician and the Resident Assistant Surgeon, above them again the junior consultant physicians and surgeons of the hospital staff, and finally the senior consultants. Little by little, as we ourselves acquired some experience and skill, we were given more and more responsibility for the care of our patients, but always under the watchful eye of our seniors. Thus did we come to gain more and more confidence in our own powers of dealing with sickness and disease by what were recognized at that time to be the best methods of treatment, and very gradually we were allowed more and more to apply these methods with the use of our own judgment and initiative. I think of the names of many eminent men under whose care I came as a medical student—Cuthbert Wallace, Nitch, Battle, Max Page, Adams, Norbury, Maybury, Turney, Cassidy, Caiger, Fisher, Hudson, Marriage, Howarth, Fairbairn, Hedley, Mennell, Mitchiner, Shattock and Dudgeon; I could multiply this list several times. The names may mean little to those who were not closely acquainted with them, but they will mean much to my contemporaries who also trained under them.

At the outbreak of the First World War in 1914 I was still a medical student. My eldest brother enlisted at once, in the middle of his undergraduate career full of brilliant promise at Balliol College, and joined a Public Schools infantry battalion of the Middlesex Regiment as a private. My second brother, by virtue of distinction he had gained in the Officer's Training

Corps at school and university, obtained a commission in the Somerset Light Infantry. I myself followed instructions from above that medical students half-way through their training should proceed to qualification so that they could serve as medical officers in the forces later on. I confess I felt some qualms about this when some of my contemporary medical students ignored these instructions and joined the army in a combatant capacity, or the navy as surgeon-probationers, but I allowed myself to be persuaded that I was following the right course. Consequently, it was not till the latter part of the war that I joined the Royal Army Medical Corps as a medical officer. After some preliminary training at Millbank, and then as a regimental medical officer attached to a battalion in camp in Staffordshire, I was sent out to France early in 1918. For a few days I was stationed at Wimereux near Boulogne, waiting to be posted to a battalion in the forward trenches, but on the very eve of my departure for the front I contracted diphtheria and was moved by ambulance to a fever hospital near by where I was placed on the 'seriously ill' list for a few weeks. But I made a satisfactory recovery, and after a short convalescent leave in England I was posted for duty at No. 8 Stationary Hospital at Wimereux where I remained on the medical staff for the rest of the war. At the time, this interlude of diphtheria seemed to be something of a calamity. Looking back, I think it might better be regarded as a fortunate episode, for a number of the medical officers who had originally accompanied me to France and were sent up to the front line did not return, or they returned with mutilating wounds.

My two brothers were not so fortunate.

Being a junior medical officer, I was allocated to one ward or another in the Stationary Hospital as the need arose, working in a capacity equivalent to a house surgeon or house physician, but with more responsibility. Thus on one occasion I had the care of patients in a special ward devoted to wounds

involving fractures of the thigh bone, on another I had charge
of penetrating chest injuries, or yet again I worked in wards of
trench fever and influenza patients. The clinical staff of the
hospital was on the whole outstandingly good. There were
some excellent surgeons (and one or two not so excellent), and
also two senior physicians of distinction, one who later became
Sir Henry Tidy (and a senior consultant at St. Thomas's
Hospital), and the other Carmalt-Jones who after the war was
appointed Professor of Medicine in the University of Otago in
New Zealand. And there was another member of the hospital
staff, one of the pathologists, who was destined to become
world-famous for his initial discovery of penicillin, Alexander
Fleming. At that time Fleming was working in close collaboration with Sir Almroth Wright on the bacterial infection of
war wounds and finding that some of the antiseptics commonly
used in their treatment were much less effective than had been
supposed. The antiseptics, they showed, might actually
interfere with the protective action of the white blood cells
of which pus is composed, for many of these cells discharged
into suppurating wounds are still capable of destroying large
numbers of the infective micro-organisms. Fleming's observations made me think that the phrase 'laudable pus' used by
surgeons of old in pre-antiseptic days was not so stupid after
all. Apart from his research work, Fleming was rather a gay
member of the officers' mess, and not averse to an occasional
practical joke. Working with such men, and largely under
their supervision, I gained valuable experience in a wide field of
clinical methods. The work imposed a fairly severe strain,
particularly during the desperate fighting of the last German
offensive of 1918 when convoys of wounded arrived in rapid
succession day and night. It was a time when man-power for
the fighting forces was becoming a serious problem, and many
of the badly wounded were lads of hardly more than eighteen
or twenty years.

The armistice came, with local celebrations in which I took part with a considerable feeling of relief after witnessing the misery and suffering of so many maimed and dying men in such concentrated numbers. But even this sense of relief came to be completely overshadowed when, a few days later, I heard of the most grievous injury that my eldest brother had suffered on armistice day itself, the more overwhelming in its effects on all of my family because, having been through the whole war in France and in many situations of great danger, he had up to then marvellously escaped safe and sound. Meanwhile, my other brother had suffered from shell-shock in 1915 after being blown up by a mine in France and had to undergo prolonged treatment in hospital. Then, towards the end of 1916, he was transferred to the Indian Army, but on his way to Madras his ship was torpedoed in the Mediterranean and he was lucky enough to be rescued by a hospital ship and landed at Alexandria. He recovered from these calamities physically, and though unimpaired in his intellectual and administrative ability or in his capacity for persistent hard work, I think they affected (as, indeed, they were bound to do) his emotional attitude towards world affairs generally. Like many of us after submergence in the almost mechanical and automatic day-by-day operations of war-time necessities, he came to the surface of peace with feelings of disillusionment.

As for me, after the armistice there followed a short period of my life of which there is a curious blank in my memory. I know I went to Cologne with the army of occupation, and I can see myself, as it were objectively but without any vivid feeling of recollection, trundling across the devastated areas of northern France and Belgium in a railway wagon labelled '20 Hommes, 8 Chevaux', and I know I was billeted for a brief while in a village called Gladbach near Cologne. But I do not recall my return journey from Germany, nor have I any conscious memory of being demobilized in 1919. Thereafter I spent a few months working at St. Thomas's Hospital and it was there that, as I have already recounted, I decided to cut myself adrift, so to speak, by seeking a completely new environment in one of the less frequented parts of the world and found myself appointed Principal Medical Officer of Sarawak in Borneo.

All the varied clinical experiences that I gained at St. Thomas's Hospital, and in France during the war, came to serve me in very good stead in Sarawak, for there I was faced with much heavier responsibilities, and without the opportunity of getting advice from specialists in the various branches of medicine and surgery. I had to engage in clinical work of all kinds, medical, surgical and obstetric, in which I had the care of patients of many races—Malays, Chinese, Indians, Europeans, Dyaks and others, ranging in status from the Rajah down to the humblest of jungle inhabitants. Further, apart from the administrative responsibility for all the Government Medical Services, including a number of medical centres in widely scattered districts as well as the Public Health Department, I had charge of a leper hospital and a ward of mentally deranged patients. Another duty of the Principal Medical Officer, as I was informed soon after my arrival in Sarawak, required attendance at the execution of criminals convicted of murder. But during my three years in the country no occasion arose for this disagreeable office—an interesting commentary on the harmonious and law-abiding relationships of the various native communities. Incidentally, the method of execution employed in those days was shooting by a firing squad, a method that had superseded the traditional operation of plunging a Malay kris down behind the collarbone straight into the heart. An unpleasant-sounding operation but no doubt one that, skilfully applied, would lead to almost instantaneous death.

When I came to Sarawak I found only one other European doctor in Kuching, and he was due to retire in a few months time. In distant parts of the country there were also two or three doctors employed by trading companies, but I only occasionally came into contact with them. Otherwise, my staff consisted of non-Europeans. Most of these did not have recognized medical qualifications that would be accepted in England, but some were extraordinarily efficient in most branches of medical practice except major surgery. There was a large non-European hospital and a small European hospital (later, I am glad to say, this segregation of hospitals was no longer maintained). There was a Scottish matron, Miss Tait, in charge of patients at the European hospital who also gave invaluable service in the non-European hospital. In personal charge of the latter was an able Chinese doctor, Swee Kim, a man of fine personality and great integrity of character; he was fated later to lose his life by drowning in a valiant attempt to save one of his friends who had got into difficulties while bathing off the coast. Then there was Tan Sim Poh, a kindly and courteous gentleman who was not only skilled in the diagnosis and treatment of medical cases but also a very able anaesthetist. The operating theatre and its equipment were under the charge of an elderly Chinese, Thian Soo, who was responsible for preparing and sterilizing all the instruments and other accessories required for each operation. The dispensary was supervised by my efficient Head Dispenser, Hon Chon Vong, who had under his direction for assistance and training a staff of younger dispensers. To assist me in the outpatient department I had an Indian doctor, Dr Chand, and with him, as also at the hospital, a company of dressers of various grades of seniority; these were a mixed lot in their racial origin—Dyaks, Chinese, Malays and Eurasians, who worked industriously and with intelligence. We used to train dressers locally, and when after some years they had become proficient in the diagnosis and routine treatment of common types of illness and injury, they were periodically drafted to small outstations to take charge of local dispensaries there. Those in charge of outstation clinics reported to me regularly by surface mail, and by wireless in the case of an emergency, and, of course, I visited them from time to time. I myself gave systematic lectures on general anatomy and physiology, and also clinical instruction during my daily rounds of visits in the wards.

All in all, in spite of the fact that the equipment of the medical services was in many respects rather primitive when I assumed my duties in 1920, and the staff inadequate in number and very few of them well qualified, the medical organization was reasonably sound. But there was a great deal to be done to improve the general standard of medical care all over Sarawak. By degrees I increased the size of the staff and organized their training by more intensive and comprehensive courses of lectures and demonstrations. Later I was able to add three more European doctors to my Department; they were Dr J. G. Reed, who had been with me at St. Thomas's Hospital, Dr O'Driscoll, a woman doctor who took on the duties of pathologist and also had the care of women and children in Kuching, and Dr Marjoribanks, who succeeded me as Principal Medical Officer when I returned to England after my three years of office. Of all my many duties, those involving major surgery were at first the most disconcerting. None of my predecessors in the Government Medical Service had any special surgical qualifications, and there was a natural reluctance on the part of the native population to submit themselves to surgical treatment. I decided to proceed with the utmost caution in this particular field of work and refused to under-take any surgery unless, after I had carefully explained the exact nature of the ailment to my patients and the exact nature of the surgical treatment required, they freely expressed their willingness to undergo an operation. I recollect very well a Chinese patient who entered hospital with a subacute obstruction of the bowel that I could easily have relieved by an abdominal operation; his condition day by day grew worse, and although I spent some time each day and explained, with the help of blackboard diagrams, precisely what was wrong and how it could be remedied, he would not countenance an operation and eventually died. Shortly after, I had another patient whose leg had been severely mauled by a crocodile and who arrived in hospital with commencing gangrene of the foot. Again I explained to him that he would inevitably die unless I amputated his leg forthwith, but again he refused to let me do this and he also died. But I eventually won respect for the achievements of surgery when one of my own dressers, Taneh, suddenly perforated an ulcer of the stomach. Now this man was a Milanau and the Milanau people were particularly suspicious of European medicine, but he himself had come to have complete confidence in me and willingly allowed me to do the only thing likely to save his life, that was to open his abdomen and repair the perforation. Not so his relatives; his aged father begged me not to operate, and his wife clutched hold of me and entreated me with tears to stay my hand. I might have wavered under the circumstances for I knew that if the operation were not successful others might lose what confidence they had in me and it would take some time to regain it. However, I was quite certain of my diagnosis and operated immediately, and fortunately the patient made an excellent recovery. The result was striking, for the details of the operation were widely broadcast by those of my staff who assisted me in carrying it out, and the native people seemed inclined to regard the whole business as akin to the miraculous. From then onwards, confidence in my surgical ability grew, and I had little difficulty in persuading those who consulted me to undergo an operation if this were needed. Looking back, I confess to a feeling of some astonishment at the variety of surgical procedures that I undertook and also at my apparent boldness in undertaking them, for they sometimes involved operations of considerable complexity. But the cases presented themselves and I had to do my best to deal with them—abdominal operations, genito-urinary surgery, difficult ortho-paedic cases, an occasional intra-cranial operation, to say nothing of other oddments such as cataract extraction, skin-grafting in severe lacerating injuries, plastic surgery for con-genital deformities, removal of tumours, and so forth. I am happy to remember that I achieved a fair measure of success in my surgery in spite of the fact that, though I had of course had some previous surgical experience, this had been rather limited in scope. But I had one great advantage in this variety of work; I had a very intimate knowledge of the anatomy of the human body, and I came to realize that with a really close familiarity with anatomical details it is possible to undertake a diversity of operations even if previous experience in specialized surgical techniques may have been somewhat limited. By contrast (and I commend this principle to those medical educationalists of today who seek to limit the time available for the preclinical subjects of the medical curriculum), however skilful a surgeon may be in the actual technique of operations, he cannot proceed very far unless he really has become well versed in topographical anatomy.

I am tempted here to make mention of one little operation which was perhaps peculiar to Sarawak in my days, a simple plastic operation that I devised and to which I used jokingly to refer as the 'Sarawak operation for lobuloplasty'. It is the custom of some of the indigenous peoples of the country to distend the lobes of their ears by perforating them and inserting into the holes wooden discs of increasing size until the lobes were extended to form long loops hanging down almost to their shoulders and weighted with heavy brass rings. When from time to time some of these men from up-country districts came to Kuching to work in a Government Department, they frequently felt sensitive and embarrassed at what they came to think of as relics of an 'uncivilized' practice and begged me to restore to them ear-lobes of normal appearance. This could be done quite simply in a few minutes with a local anaesthetic. Incidentally, they were the only cases in which I regularly charged a fee—one Singapore dollar. I used to collect these dollars in a hospital fund, and each year they contributed to an accumulated sum of modest fees that on occasion I charged a few of the richer Chinese merchants for surgical treatment, and all this we expended on a grand feast for the medical staff of the hospital, an annual occasion for our mutual enjoyment and merriment.

The remarkable variety of my medical work in Sarawak gave it an interest and a mental stimulus that I found quite absorbing, an intellectual adventure that paralleled the adventures of my jungle explorations. If I had a major operation to perform, I did this first thing in the morning before the heat of the day had risen to an uncomfortable level for work in gown, mask and surgical gloves (for in my time there were no air conditioning plants in Sarawak). Then followed a session with out-patients and visits to the hospital wards. The early afternoon I commonly used for the instruction of my staff by lectures and demonstrations and, should there be an occasion for it, for carrying out a post-mortem examination. At regular intervals I visited the mental ward, and also the leper hospital some few miles from Kuching. These last two duties gave me a sense of frustration, for there was almost nothing I could do for the mentally ill patients and very little for the lepers. It is difficult enough to enter into the minds of the mentally afflicted when you can talk with a common language; it is next to impossible when you can only converse in a language that is not your own unless, indeed, you have achieved a very high degree of fluency. But I could give the sympathetic word in Malay and, even more important, the sympathetic touch, and it is remarkable to me that some of the patients who seemed to be suffering from the most intractable delusions did make improvement and, on occasion, an apparent recovery. No doubt the prolonged rest and care that these poor people received, and the continual encouragement from those who attended them combined with a freedom from personal responsibilities, helped them on to a readjustment from their mental aberrations and so led to improvement and sometimes to a restitution of their normal mentality.

For leprosy we did not have the sulphone compounds that today are often so effective in its treatment. We had to rely on injections of a rather crude form of chaulmoogra oil, a treatment that was not only painful in its administration but was very uncertain in its results. But my visits to the leper hospital were something of an inspiration to me because of the amazing cheerfulness and courage of the patients, even of those most severely afflicted. They showed all degrees in the progress of the disease, some in quite early stages with the characteristic nodules of skin infiltration, others with the gross deformities produced by erosion of fingers to mere stumps, some almost blind with corneal opacities, and others near to death with the complications that set in at the last phases of the infection. Yet always they greeted me with fervent handshakes and smiles of gratitude for what had been done to help them. This general atmosphere of cheerfulness pervading the leper hospital was in large measure due to the devoted care and attention the patients received from a little old lady, Miss Cubitt, who lived with them, and I find it difficult adequately to express my admiration for the way in which she sacrificed herself completely in her love for these sick and dying people. The phrase 'saintliness of character' is sometimes used rather extravagantly, but I think it strictly applied to Miss Cubitt. She was a member of the Staff of the S.P.G. Mission in Sarawak, and having had some training and experience in nursing she decided to abandon

her usual missionary occupations in Kuching and to isolate
herself with the lepers in their jungle settlement. She not only
attended to the daily dressing of their sores and the administration of such medicines as might alleviate their sufferings, by the
sheer force of her sympathetic personality she inspired them all
with a deep affection for her and with a superlative moral
courage.

While, in spite of limited facilities, I felt fairly confident in
my ability to cope with routine medical duties, I always had
lurking in the back of my mind the anxiety of an outbreak of
an epidemic of some sort in Sarawak. I knew that, some years
before my arrival in the country, there had been an outbreak of
cholera, and many fatalities had followed the world-wide
pandemic of influenza after the First World War. If an epidemic occurred again, I could not see how with my inadequate
staff I should be able to deal with it successfully. Each week
when the ship from Singapore arrived, I used to go on board
and carefully examine every immigrant, mostly Chinese. If
any of them showed symptoms of an infection they were
immediately transferred to a quarantine ward and kept there
until I was able to satisfy myself that the infection was not of a
serious nature. But I was lucky. Only on one occasion did the
threat of an epidemic show itself. Shortly after a ship-load of
passengers had left Miri in northern Sarawak on their few days'
voyage down the coast to Kuching, I received a wireless
message reporting a case of smallpox where they had embarked.
I had to act quickly and, taking possession of two empty
bungalows near the mouth of the Kuching river, I rapidly
converted them into a quarantine station where I could
disembark the passengers, vaccinate them, and lodge them
until the quarantine period was over. In the event, however, it
turned out to be unnecessary, for two days after their arrival I
received another wireless message from Miri reporting a wrong
diagnosis; the suspected case of smallpox had been recognized

to be an unusually severe case of chickenpox, a diagnostic mistake that can sometimes be made even by an experienced clinician.

Among my various responsibilities were those concerned with medico-legal problems, whether there might be evidence of insanity in a case of homicide (there was in fact definite evidence of a disturbed state of mind in the only two cases on which I had to give a medical opinion), whether a wound had been self-inflicted or not, or how long had death occurred before a dead body was found. The most horrific experience of this kind that I had to deal with was, I think, the most loathsome duty I ever had to undertake in the whole of my medical career. A Chinese rubber planter who lived alone a few miles from Kuching in an isolated small tumble-down wooden bungalow, indeed hardly more than a shack, was reported to have hanged himself three days previously, and it must be remembered that decomposition after death proceeds very rapidly in a humid tropical climate. I went out to examine the situation and as I began to approach the bungalow I was assaulted by the foul smell of putrefaction. Walking up the garden path to the steps of the verandah, the stench became still more penetrating and I suddenly caught sight of some maggots crawling on the path. When I did reach the verandah I was faced with a most appalling sight; hanging from a beam was a bloated semblance of a man entirely encased from head to foot in a teeming mass of squirming maggots—no part of the body itself was visible. The foetid smell was overwhelming, and with the utterly nauseating appearance of such a grotesquely distorted human figure, as it were modelled in myriads of ceaseless writhings, it was all too much for me. I vomited. What was I to do? There was only one thing I could do. After removing such articles of furniture and other things that were worth removing, I fetched some cans of petrol that I poured over the verandah and other parts of the bungalow and set fire to it. The whole bungalow with its horrid contents went up in flames, maggots and all. There was no need to carry out a post-mortem on the body to ascertain the cause of death; indeed, it would have been physically impossible to attempt such a revolting examination. I suppose few laymen realize what offensively unpleasant tasks a medical man is required to undertake from time to time, particularly in medico-legal work, but I can hardly imagine anything more unpleasant than this particular episode.

The epidemic diseases in Sarawak included (apart from leprosy, amoebic dysentery and certain other afflictions such as beri-beri, fungoid skin infections and trachoma) malaria, filariasis, hook-worm infestation, tuberculosis and yaws. Malaria was common enough up-country but, to my surprise, not a serious problem in the more populated centres in spite of the prevalence of the *Anopheles* mosquito that carries the malarial parasite. Of course we all used to sleep under mosquito nets which no doubt lessened the chances of infection, but I myself never took any prophylactic doses of quinine even when travelling in jungle areas up-country. Filariasis was also not as common as I had expected, though I had a few cases of elephantiasis resulting from this infection, which I dealt with surgically. Hook-worm infestation was prevalent, particularly among the Malays who had not learnt the danger of drinking water likely to be contaminated with the eggs of this parasite. Tuberculosis, particularly rife in the crowded quarters of the Chinese 'bazaars', posed a more serious problem.

Yaws was very common among the indigenous people up-country; in some parts of Sarawak about one-third of the population suffered from it. It is a disease somewhat like syphilis in its manifestations and conveyed by a similar sort of micro-organism. But it is not a venereal disease; the infection is conveyed by contact probably through skin abrasions. Fortunately, yaws was very amenable to treatment by

intravenous injections of arsenical compounds of the salvarsan
group. In fact, a single injection gave most dramatic results
and often appeared to lead to a complete cure, though repeated
treatment may in some cases be needed to ensure the total
eradication of the infection. In order to deal with this endemic
disease, from time to time I used to travel long distances into
the interior of Sarawak with large quantities of Neosalvarsan
and packing-cases filled with bottles of distilled water for making
up the injection fluid. I visited one 'long house' after another
strung at intervals beside the rivers and treated hundreds
of individuals, men, women and children. These expeditions
were full of interest for me, for I often had occasion to stay the
night in some of these houses, and to meet and get to know
many of the hundred or more individuals who lived in them.
The rapid and remarkable effect of the injections for yaws
seemed to be regarded by the native people as a powerful sort
of magic, and it was largely by these expeditions that I came to
acquire an entirely undeserved reputation as a quite phenomenal
'medicine man'. As a result, it was up-river in the Simanggang
area of Sarawak that I graduated as a fellow-member of the
community of Sea Dyaks with all due ceremony, including
the sprinkling over myself of the blood of a fresh-killed fowl
and the ceremonial drinking of a bowl of the potent rice-
spirit called borak. The ritual of presenting the borak was
performed by a young Dyak girl; clad in little more than a
sarong and decorated with bangles and hair ornaments, she
knelt before me and held the bowl to my lips, compelling me
to drink its contents with no pause for breath. Then, lighting
in her mouth a cigarette that she had prepared with native
tobacco rolled in dried banana leaf, she placed it in my mouth.
There followed a feast with all the inhabitants of the long house,
the mainstay of the meal being small lumps of boiled pork and
handfuls of boiled rice washed down with more borak. Some
of their symbolic dances were accompanied by the beating of

gongs of graded size and tone. The most sensational of these dances were those of young 'warriors' in their war coats adorned with hornbill feathers, and with their shields and parangs and plumed head-dresses. So it went on far into the night. My Dyak girl, who now sat beside me, had seemed demure and shy when she first approached me with her offerings of borak and cigarette. But mellowing with the excitement of the merry-making she nestled up against me with a warm intimacy that grew warmer as the hours flowed on. Her name, I remember, was Madu, the Dyak word for 'honey', appropriate enough for the sweetness of her youthful charm.

It was on this occasion that I came to be known among the Dyaks as the Tuan Manang B'sai, which means the Great Chief of the Witch Doctors, and in order to consummate my initiation I allowed myself to be tattooed on my shoulders with the insignia common to many of the indigenous peoples of Borneo, patterns of rosette form that are stylizations of the flower and fruit of the mangosteen. It may be that I tend now to over-emphasize incidents of this sort, and perhaps unduly to sentimentalize them. But I freely admit that the badges of honour that I carry permanently engraved on my shoulders give me as much pride and pleasure as some of the academic honours that happened to come my way later. Understandably, I suppose, for they represent to me the culmination of three years of intensive and happy work among all the many different peoples of Sarawak.

CHAPTER 3

ON BECOMING AN ANATOMIST

IN 1923, towards the end of my three years contract as
Principal Medical Officer of Sarawak, I seriously considered
the idea of renewing my appointment with the intention of
making a permanent career there. I had come very near to a
definite decision to do so, when two unexpected events
occurred that turned my thoughts in another direction. I
received a letter from my old Professor at St. Thomas's
Hospital, F. G. Parsons, telling me that the Chair of Anatomy
at St. Bartholomew's Hospital Medical School was about to
become vacant, and suggesting that I should apply for the post.
I demurred in my reply for it seemed to me that I had too few
qualifications for so elevated an academic position. I pointed
out that I had had no more than one year's experience as a
demonstrator of anatomy, and, though I had completed two
scientific papers before I went to Sarawak (one on the cranial
characters of the Eskimo and the other on certain granulations
on the membranes of the brain concerned with the circulation
of the cerebrospinal fluid), these were rather trivial contributions in the field of anatomical research. On the other hand, I
had to my credit a considerable administrative experience from
supervising the Government Medical Service of Sarawak; I
had kept in touch by correspondence with eminent anatomists
of the day in England and elsewhere, acquainting them from
time to time with my observations on some of the Bornean
animals; and I also had the Fellowship of the Royal College of
Surgeons which in those days was regarded as an important
qualification for a Professor of Anatomy at a London Medical
school. Yet I could not persuade myself that these were assets

of sufficient worth to justify an application for the Chair. Then I received further letters from Parsons, and also from Elliot Smith who was the professor of Anatomy at University College, London, strongly urging me to apply for the post, and I felt less hesitant in submitting to their insistent requests. The other event was much more personal. Just about that time a lady, Mrs Giddey, and her young daughter, who were making a leisurely journey in the East on their way back to England, were persuaded by friends to interrupt their stay in Singapore and pay a visit to Sarawak. They arrived in Kuching but were there no more than a few days before leaving to renew their travels, and I myself only had the opportunity of meeting them for a few hours. But I very much wanted to meet them again, or, I should more truly say, to meet *her*. In order to satisfy this feeling of urgency, I had to act very rapidly after their departure, and I cabled to an acquaintance of mine in Singapore asking him to make discreet enquiries about their immediate destination. Hearing that they were shortly due to reach Hong Kong, I applied for six weeks' leave (which in any case was then due to me) and followed them to China. It was a short but supremely happy interlude, long enough for Freda and myself to get closely acquainted to the extent that there grew between us a deeply affectionate understanding, and we parted in our different directions leaving me with the determination to be with her again as soon as she returned to England.

The two events to which I have referred outweighed any previous inclination to prolong my working life in Sarawak, joyous though this had been for me. I later submitted my candidature for the Chair of Anatomy at Bart's and, to my surprise and pleasure, my application was successful. I returned to England in the late summer of 1923, met Freda when she reached London, became formally engaged to her in October, and we were married at the end of the year. Thus started a new chapter in my life. Reasonably enough, in view of my very limited academic experience, the electors to the Chair did not immediately grant me the full professorship; they gave me for a probationary period the less elevated status of a Reader, though I had the full responsibilities of a Professor in the administrative, teaching and research duties required for the director of an anatomical department at one of the largest medical schools of London University. But after three years I was promoted to the professorship, with an increase of my salary from £800 to £1,000 a year for which I was very grateful; even in those days it was by no means easy to marry and bring up a family on the smaller salary, and for a time we had to live very modestly indeed. Our first daughter, Joan, was born while we were living in a small flat in London, and in 1927 we were able to buy a country house in the village of Digswell in Hertfordshire where, in 1928, our second daughter, Pauline, arrived.

The years of family life at Digswell were years of great gladness for me, and the aroma of happiness that they left behind still permeates the matrix of my mind. But I passed through a period of worrying anxiety at first because I did not find it easy to adjust myself so abruptly to the combined demands of domestic and academic responsibilities. Particularly the latter, for these, to begin with, were very exacting. But I was fortunate to have an intimate personal friend who gave me much kindly advice as my confidant and mentor, and my mood of apprehensive tension passed as rapidly as it overtook me. Looking back, I realize how much I owed to my friend for his help during this short period of stress.

I was at first somewhat surprised to discover how primitive were the accommodation and facilities of the Department of Anatomy at Bart's when I started work there in 1924, though they could no doubt be paralleled by some other university departments at that time. There was, of course, a dissecting-room—placed oddly enough, in a block right in the centre of the hospital. A gallery above this room contained a number of anatomical models, and dissected specimens in bottles for teaching purposes. Below the dissecting-room, in a dank-smelling sort of dungeon, was the mortuary where cadavers for dissection were embalmed and stored; presiding over this was an aged man with a tobacco-stained moustache and a beery breath and, as I recall, not infrequently a beerily unsteady manner of walking. He it was who embalmed the bodies and I remember that with some feelings of repulsion I occasionally found him eating his lunch down below, surrounded by his handiwork. But the poor man had nowhere else to go, for there was no such thing as a technician's common-room in the Medical School. He was skilful enough in the technique of embalming, but I was always filled with qualms as to his ability to observe with due care all the strict regulations regarding the acceptance of human cadavers for dissection, and the disposal thereafter of the remains for proper burial.

My own personal accommodation in the Anatomy Department consisted of a tiny office that found room for little more than a desk, and, leading off from the gallery of the dissecting-room, a research laboratory. At least it was called a research laboratory if by that term is understood a small room containing a laboratory bench with a sink, a microscope of simple construction, and an old-fashioned microtome for cutting sections of tissues embedded in paraffin wax. I had little more in the way of equipment, no secretary, no laboratory technician to assist me, and none of the more elaborate apparatus regarded today as essential for anatomical research. Thus, in trying to accomplish some of my early research work I had to do everything myself, including my own 'bottle-washing'. This will perhaps surprise young anatomists of today who are provided with technicians, cleaners, secretarial assistance, research microscopes of modern design, workshop facilities, photographic equipment, and may be with more elaborate apparatus such as calculating machines and electron microscopes. But at least I had one advantage; in having to do everything myself I mastered the basic laboratory methods very thoroughly and thus came to recognize (perhaps more clearly than some of my successors) the snags and pitfalls that may frustrate and prevent technically good results. I also learned more quickly how to apply elementary techniques intelligently and economically so that when in later academic appointments I did have laboratory and other assistants I was in a good position to instruct them and supervise their work to suit my particular objectives.

With the meagre facilities provided for me at Bart's I was not able to develop my programme of research on the scale I would have liked, and, in any case, I was kept very hard at work with my teaching duties. Apart from one (more or less) 'full-time' demonstrator, I had only part-time teaching assistants who were young surgeons aspiring to become candidates for staff appointments at the hospital when these should become vacant. I myself gave four formal lectures a week and two or three revision classes, as well as special classes for those students preparing for the Primary Fellowship examination of the Royal College of Surgeons. And in addition to all this I spent some hours each day with my students supervising their practical dissections and testing their knowledge by periodical discussions with them. In my formal lectures I had to deal with every aspect of anatomy: its general principles, gross topographical anatomy with particular emphasis on clinical applications, embryology, neurological anatomy, radiological anatomy, and so forth. Having to grapple with so wide a range of subjects in my lecture courses, I naturally came to acquire a wide knowledge of the literature dealing with them. The familiarity I thus gained with current advances in all branches of anatomical science, as well as in related fields of biology and physiology, stood me in good stead later on because of the possible bearing of these subjects on those in which I came to specialize. But those early years at Bart's demanded a great deal of hard work that commonly kept me busy into the late hours of the night.

My immediate colleagues at Bart's were genial and helpful: Lovatt Evans was the professor of physiology, ready in advice as to the experimental methods that I wanted to apply in some of my research problems. Soon after my arrival he was elected to the Fellowship of the Royal Society and later he transferred to the Chair of Physiology at University College, London, where he had a distinguished career. He was followed by Hartridge, a man of buoyant temperament who, like myself, did not get on very well with the Dean of the Medical School. No doubt the Dean of that time was able as an administrator, but he had a somewhat irascible disposition, apt to flare up tactlessly with unnecessary vehemence when he supposed (quite wrongly, I think) that we were not carrying out our duties in accordance with traditional requirements, and unreasonably suspicious of any innovations that we sought to introduce into the curriculum. I therefore used to ignore his tendency to inference and to proceed with my own ideas for improving the organization of my department. Our relations were on the whole not very friendly. With a few exceptions also, the senior members of the clinical staff seemed to me to be rather aloof in their attitude towards the preclinical departments. Of course they were all a good deal older than myself and for this reason alone, perhaps, we did not have very much in common with each other. But the senior surgeon, Sir Holburt Waring, in spite of a certain abruptness of manner and gruffness of speech, was always sympathetic to me in some of the difficulties I encountered from time to time in connexion with my work. It was he, I fancy, who put forward my claims for the Triennial Prize of the Royal College of Surgeons, in the form of a medal embossed with the portrait of John

Hunter, which I received in 1924. I was naturally proud of this first medal awarded to me; I recollect that I was asked whether I would elect to receive a gold medal, or a bronze medal and fifty pounds. I chose the latter partly, I suspect, because I wanted to display this coveted prize on my mantel-piece at home (a gold medal would need to be held secure in the vaults of my bank), but mainly because at that time I needed the money for family expenses. Two of the senior pathologists I came to know well, Mervyn Gordon and Bernard Spilsbury. It so happened that Mervyn Gordon was at that time enquiring into the possible routes whereby the virus of encephalitis reaches the brain, and he was led to suspect that it does so through the nasal cavities. He therefore asked me whether any such pathways of access to the brain could be demonstrated anatomically. This led me to an experimental investigation, and I was able to show that innocuous solutions dropped into the nose of rabbits did indeed reach the surface of the brain within a few hours by tracking up along the sheaths of the olfactory nerves and thus entering the intracranial cavity quite rapidly. I was interested to find, a few weeks after the publication of my paper, that I was attacked quite vigorously by the Anti-vivisection Society for carrying out such simple experiments that caused no distress whatever to my rabbits and which supplied quite useful information on the mode of access by virus infections affecting the brain in human patients. Spilsbury I got to know through meeting him from time to time at the staff luncheon table in the hospital refectory. He was not an easy man to get closely acquainted with, for he was reserved in temperament and modest to a degree of shyness. But we established very friendly relations because of common interests. He was then at the height of his career as a medico-legal expert, in those days undoubtedly the most distinguished pathologist in this field of work. He was once described as the 'perfect witness' in legal trials involving medical evidence because he was cautious in statement, tended to understate his case for the prosecution, and gave his evidence with a simplicity and directness that rarely failed to impress his legal colleagues. In 1924 he was working on the Crowborough murder, and I was privileged to visit him from time to time in his laboratory and study the microscopic sections of the tissues of the murdered girl demonstrating the evidence of injuries resulting from a violent attack before her death. But Spilsbury had a tragic life; one son was killed in the bombing of St. Thomas's Hospital in 1940 (he had previously been a student of mine), and he lost his other son who died of tuberculosis in 1945. He was so deeply affected by these bereavements that he terminated his own life in 1947.

Some of the younger surgeons at Bart's, more my con-temporaries in age, I came to know very well, for several of them worked under my supervision as part-time demonstrators of anatomy. Always conscientious in their teaching duties, they became my intimate friends and collaborators, and I look back with great pleasure on the companionship they gave me. They were also friends of my family and from time to time visited us in our country home in Digswell for a meal or a game of tennis. Most of them in later years achieved distinction in one or another of the fields of surgery, becoming senior consultants on the staffs of the big hospitals in London and elsewhere, and two of them later received a knighthood in recognition of their outstanding ability.

It is interesting to look back on those days when, apart from the professor, the routine teaching in the anatomy departments of most medical schools was largely carried out by young surgeons who acted as part-time demonstrators and were waiting their chances of promotion to staff appointments in surgery. Indeed, their chances were not very favourable unless they had served their two or three years of apprentice-ship as anatomy demonstrators. They received a salary of only £150 a year on their first appointment, and no doubt the medical schools found this a very inexpensive way of financing anatomical teaching. It was a parsimonious custom to say the least of it, and it had serious disadvantages. For one thing, the surgeon demonstrators, naturally enough, tended to focus the attention of students on those aspects of topographical anatomy that are important to the surgical specialist, in spite of the fact that only a very small proportion of the medical students whom they taught were ever likely to make a career in major surgery. For another thing, they had no time to take part in research activities that today are regarded as an important part of the duties of the staff of preclinical departments. But funds were not then usually available for the appointment of full-time demonstrators in adequate number, and medical schools were compelled to carry on as best they could with poorly paid part-time assistants.

In 1930 my old professor at St. Thomas's Hospital Medical School retired, and I was invited to succeed to the professorial chair there. I readily accepted the invitation, for this appointment offered substantial advantages. It provided a modest increase in salary; I welcomed the prospect of returning to my own hospital where I should be working among old friends of the preclinical and clinical departments, many of whom had been my contemporaries when I was a student; I had there a department pleasantly compact and better equipped than the department at Bart's, including a more useful research laboratory for experimental work; I had a competent full-time demonstrator to assist me; and at last I had to myself a laboratory technician to help me with my research programmes.

My immediate colleague as professor of physiology at St. Thomas's was John Mellanby, distinguished for his work on digestive enzymes. As I have already mentioned, he had taught me physiology when I was a medical student. And here I must confess that I found myself in rather a curious position to which it was not easy at first to adapt myself. For, while still at an early age, I had reached an academic position that made me equivalent in status to many older men who had been my teachers and masters in my student career. But I need not have felt any awkwardness about this because, although I naturally did not feel equal to them in experience and distinction, they certainly did their best to make me feel I was their equal and they were always ready to give me encouragement and kindly advice. In this connexion I think particularly of the professor of anatomy at University College, Elliot Smith, and J. P. Hill, professor of embryology at the same institution. I frequently used to visit them to discuss problems that were engaging my attention, and they allowed me to make use of research material and equipment that were not available to me in my own department, and to obtain the assistance of their highly trained microphotographer and anatomical artist. Elliot Smith was one of the most distinguished British anatomists of the time, a man of exceptionally wide interests ranging from the comparative anatomy and evolution of the brain to Egyptology. Before his appointment to University College he had been the professor of anatomy at Cairo University and had made extensive studies of ancient Egyptian tombs; it was on the basis of these studies that he developed the thesis of a wide diffusion of culture from the Nile Valley extending over most parts of the world—even to the old Mayan civilization of the New World. The thesis came in for vigorous criticism from some ethnologists who maintained that he carried his conclusions too far beyond the evidence on which he sought to prove them. The consensus of opinion today is that he did indeed overrate the validity of the evidence for such a wide diffusion of culture, but at least he drew attention to the importance of the factor of diffusion in early times to which ethnologists had not given sufficient attention.

Another distinguished anatomist who was also very helpful

to me in advice and encouragement was Sir Arthur Keith, Conservator of the Hunterian Museum in the Royal College of Surgeons, whose primary interest at that time was the study of the fossil evidence for human evolution. Unfortunately he and Elliot Smith were at intellectual loggerheads with each other which found expression in acrimonious disputes in certain scientific journals. These found their focus in a somewhat unseemly wrangle over the famous Piltdown skull that many years later was shown to be the product of an unscrupulous archaeological forgery (for the details of the exposure of this forgery see Chapter 9). Actually, Keith proved to be more in the right in this argumentative discussion even though he did accept the skull as a genuine fossil of great antiquity. But they were of a very different temperament—Elliot Smith more aggressive and much more skilful in polemical debate, and Keith of a gentler nature and thus disinclined to stand up to his formidable opponent. Consequently, to the looker-on in this war of words Elliot Smith appeared to be on the winning side. But this is a common pattern in the interchange of controversial and opposing opinions that appear in print. It is far better, as I have advised my junior colleagues who might be tempted to 'answer back' in the correspondence columns of a journal, and more dignified, to ignore polemical attacks on their stated opinions, unless such attacks include a deliberate misrepresentation of their views by erroneous statements or by misquotation. It is all too easy for the artful, and perhaps not too scrupulous, controversialist to distort the opinions of his opponent by oblique innuendoes and by quotations of statements isolated from their context. I had this unhappy experience imposed on myself on one occasion and, though my own statements were subsequently vindicated, at the time it made me think of Cowper's line in his verses on 'Conversation'—'A noisy man is always in the right.'

In the early years of my career as an anatomist, the attention of my contemporaries was mainly directed to purely descriptive studies of the details of structures in the human body and their variations, and also descriptive studies of human and other mammalian embryos and their development. J. P. Hill of University College, London, Bryce of Glasgow, Fawcett of Bristol, Wilson of Cambridge, and Frazer of St. Mary's Hospital Medical School, were the leading embryologists. The study of the earliest stages of the development of the human embryo was particularly important, of course, but at that time very little material was available for such investigations. Other anatomists interested themselves in physical anthropology of the traditional type, recording measurements of the human skull and skeleton either of modern races of mankind, or of fossil material of palaeolithic man and collections of mediaeval skeletons preserved in ossuaries. This somewhat pedestrian kind of study was useful, but it did not advance the science of anatomy very far. For example, the assumption that the history of racial origins and diversification could be unravelled by noting small differences in the shape of the skull and so forth proved to be unfounded since nothing was known of the hereditary basis of such differences or of their relation to different environmental influences. Such fallacies were inherent in the voluminous works of statisticians who began to apply their statistical methods to the study of biological problems—a branch of statistics called biometrics. One of the pioneers in this field was Karl Pearson of University College, London. But neither he, nor many younger members of his school, were versed in biological principles, and the results of their studies were therefore often misleading and open to misinterpretation. Nevertheless, they tended to develop a rather arrogant attitude towards those anatomists who were interested in physical anthropology and who were not primarily statisticians. For example, my old professor, Parsons, had made a careful and systematic study of the variations in form of the human thigh bone, based on measurements of material examined in the post-mortem room. Karl Pearson had made a similar study of the human thigh bone based on the skeletal remains of mediaeval populations disinterred from crypts of London churches and elsewhere, and in an extensive monograph he constantly referred to Parsons' work in such critical phraseology that could only be described as deliberate vituperation. In fact, Parsons' work was by far the more valuable since it was based on the thigh bones of individuals of whom he knew the age, sex, the body proportions during life, the medical history, and so forth. Karl Pearson's work was based on thigh bones of unknown individuals whose age, sex and other characteristics could only be approximately assumed and he could not make the necessary allowance for shrinkage and other deformations that would affect bones so long deposited in damp ossuaries. I mention this as another example of the futility of polemical discussions in scientific monographs. The undignified criticisms by Karl Pearson certainly affected Parsons deeply, but neither of them lived to see the work of this biometrical school come under the devastating fire of later statisticians using improved statistical techniques, and demonstrating that some of Karl Pearson's biometrical work was of questionable value. But Karl Pearson was a man of a somewhat contentious temperament, and during his life time other investigators were similarly treated to his quite unnecessarily harsh criticisms.

Some of my professorial colleagues at the London Medical Schools did not very actively engage in any research, though they earned reputations for their teaching or administrative abilities. William Wright of the London Hospital was one of the group; him I came to know very well when we were both examiners for the Royal College of Surgeons, and I once accompanied him to Toronto to examine for the Primary Fellowship of the College—the first time that this examination

was held abroad. Wright was an able Dean of his Medical
School, a man with a genial twinkle in his eyes and with a fund
of good stories; in appearance he used to remind me of some
Dickensian character—particularly when, on attending an
evening function, he arrived in a black cloak over his evening
dress, a top hat perched on his mass of fuzzy hair, and a long
gold-headed stick in his hand. He had done little research of
importance, and I think his most interesting work was an
anatomical study of the skeletal remains of the Princes in the
Tower that were examined when the urn containing them was
opened for inspection in 1933. The results of this study by
Wright and L. E. Tanner were published by the London
Society of Antiquaries in 1935. Briefly, Wright demonstrated
that the bones and teeth were certainly those of two children,
and that the state of their development indicated with a high
degree of probability that the elder (presumably Edward V)
was about twelve or thirteen years of age at the time of his
death, and the younger (presumably Richard, Duke of York)
about ten or eleven. This clearly provided strong evidence
that they died before the Battle of Bosworth in 1485 and thus
added confirmation to the opinion held by several historians
that Richard III was responsible for their murder, and not (as
some other historians had suggested) his successor Henry VII.
Incidentally, it has seemed curious to me that Josephine Tey, in
her engaging detective novel, *The Daughter of Time*, which
attempts to solve retrospectively the historical problem of the
Princes in the Tower and was published in 1951, makes no
reference to the evidence of William Wright's anatomical
studies, nor does her fictitious detective in this novel lay
sufficient stress on the Bill of Attainder issued by Henry VII in
which, among the list of misdoings attributed to Richard III,
specific mention is made of the killing of innocent children
(almost certainly a reference to the two little princes).

Another of my colleagues in London at the time when I was

at Bart's was Herbert Woollard who was then a lecturer in Anatomy at University College. Woollard was a close personal friend, partly because of our common interest in certain anatomical problems, partly because we were for a few years both medical officers in the University of London Officer's Training Corps, and partly because we enjoyed companionship on occasional walking tours either in England or abroad. He was a man of wide knowledge and a brilliant conversationalist. He had spent a year in the United States at Johns Hopkins University, and there engaged in modern methods of anatomical research by experimental techniques. Following his return to England he wrote an eventful book on *Recent Advances in Anatomy* in which he laid much stress on the importance of experimentation in anatomical research. This book did not find favour with some of the senior anatomists of the time in England whose work was to a large extent merely descriptive and observational, and who seemed to think that some of the recent advances to which he referred did not properly come within the scope of the subject of anatomy. But it seemed to me that they did not realize that in the past experimental studies had quite commonly been employed by anatomists. Did not William Harvey, in his great experimental work on the circulation of the blood published in 1628, entitle his dissertation *Exercitatio Anatomica de Motu Cordis et Sanguinis*? And for a very long time afterwards no clear distinction was made between the subjects of anatomy and physiology. It was no doubt the renewal of interest in evolutionary studies, following Darwin's exposition of Natural Selection, that focussed the attention of anatomists on purely morphological investigations to the virtual exclusion of experimental techniques. In fact, Woollard's book initiated what may be truly called a renaissance in anatomy in this country, and from that time onwards the recognized scope of the subject of anatomy became widened to more proper dimensions. Woollard later went to the University of Sidney as Professor of Anatomy, then returned to succeed me at Bart's, and was finally appointed to the Chair of Anatomy at University College that had been vacated by Elliot Smith on his retirement. Unhappily, his tenure of office at University College did not last long, for at the age of forty-nine he died with great suddenness in 1939 from a coronary thrombosis at the end of what proved to be his last lecture to his students.

Those colleagues and friends that I have mentioned were only a few among the many with whom I had close relationships in the early part of my career as an anatomist. But they stand out very vividly in my memory of this period. There was one other anatomist of distinction whom I should mention, not because he was an immediate colleague of mine in London, but because his early lectures and writings played an important part in directing my inclinations towards an anatomical vocation. This was Frederic Wood Jones. He had a varied career which he began as a medical officer in a little island of the Cocos-Keeling Atoll (incidentally in 1836 the first coral atoll to be visited by Charles Darwin), and on his return to England he published a remarkable book on *Coral and Atolls*. In his later anatomical work he devoted much of his attention to the influence of arboreal life in the preliminary phases of human evolution, and his comparative anatomical studies were wide and detailed. But he was unorthodox in many of his ideas, and became a pronounced and often too vehement anti-Darwinian. In spite of this, his expositions, whether strictly scientific or popular in nature, were stimulating and pleasingly provocative, and he had a most attractive style in the presentation of his views so that his articles and books came to be widely read and discussed. Because of their capacity for popularization of technical studies, Wood Jones, Arthur Keith and Elliot Smith came to be regarded as a sort of triumvirate of the anatomical world after the First World War.

There were indeed other distinguished British anatomists who were their contemporaries, some of them with perhaps even greater claims to academic distinction, but I doubt whether many of them were as inspired or as inspiring in their teaching and writings as those three. They had many things in common: each of them preceded the heights of his anatomical career by travels in what we sometimes called 'foreign parts'—Keith in Malaysia, Elliot Smith in Egypt, and Wood Jones in the Cocos Islands; they all excelled in the brilliance of their expositions whether in lecture halls or in their publications; they all spread their interests far afield from orthodox anatomy; and they all made exciting a subject at that time regarded by many students as dull and static. Novel interpretations, stimulating hypotheses and fertile suggestions sparkled from their minds, and though some of these later proved to be faulty and too insecurely founded on the facts then available, they were certainly thought-provoking at the time. I know that a number of young anatomists who were my contemporaries in the nineteen-twenties had been stirred to embark on an anatomical career because of the enthusiasm engendered by these three anatomists, and a number of them came to achieve very considerable distinction in their work. Scientists of imaginative and exploring mind commonly feel impelled to formulate hypotheses; many of them may later prove to be untenable, but they nevertheless do play an essential part in promoting the advancement of their subject. I sometimes think that, when those who are too prone to harp on the mistakes of their predecessors indulge in unnecessary disparagement, this is a sign of scientific immaturity, for they tend not to view such mistakes in their historical perspective.

As the publications of these three anatomists, which I assiduously read in my student days, ranged over the fields of comparative anatomy, human evolution and neurology, it is perhaps not surprising that my own interests became focussed on the same themes. In later years I engaged my attention mainly on experimental studies of the nervous system, but, apart from occasional diversions into other problems of current concern, I first concentrated my research activities on detailed studies of some of the inhabitants of the Bornean forests, particularly the tree-shrews and the little tarsiers, of both of which I had made considerable collections while in Sarawak. From exploring the jungles of Borneo where they live I now began to explore the anatomy of these interesting small mammals.

As I have already indicated, the tree-shrews (which had for a long time been grouped in zoological classifications with insectivores such as the hedgehog, mole and ground-shrew) were by some anatomists regarded as primitive Primates akin to the lemurs mainly on the basis of certain structural features of the skull and skeleton. But this interpretation had not been widely accepted. I made extended studies of the skull of tree-shrews, I dissected in great detail their internal anatomy, and I made a particularly careful examination of their brain. The results of all these studies were very illuminating to me, for they made it abundantly clear that in many details of their skeletal structure, their musculature, their visceral organs, and, above all, their brain, the tree-shrews are certainly more closely allied to the lemurs than to any of the insectivores, and that they should therefore be more logically grouped in a system of zoological classification within the order of the Primates than in the order of the Insectivora. This conclusion came to final agreement in a standard work on the classification of mammals published in 1945 by the outstanding American authority on the subject, Dr G. G. Simpson, when he placed the tree-shrews in a common group with the lower Primates, the lemurs. However, it did not find universal agreement at the time, and there are still a few zoologists who are reluctant to accord a primate status to the tree-shrews because of some of the primitive characters that they still retain in their anatomical structure. But even these few dissidents agree that, if the tree-shrews are not, properly speaking, Primates, they occupy a position that is, as it were, intermediate between mammals of the insectivore type and the lower Primates. And the fossil evidence that has accumulated over the years makes it fairly clear that the earliest representatives of the Primates that came into existence about fifty million years ago must have been rather similar to the tree-shrews that still inhabit the tropical forests of the Far East.

The tarsier (its official name is *Tarsius spectrum*) is a little creature of very curious appearance. It is arboreal and nocturnal in habit, has astonishingly large eyes and also large, mobile ears, and its hind-limbs are greatly elongated for use in leaping from branch to branch. It had never at that time been seen in zoological gardens and was supposedly a rare species. But I found in Sarawak that it is not really rare, for it can easily be found provided one looks for it in the right terrain, that is, among the trees of lowland jungle. The scientific interest of the tarsier lay in the dispute about its relationship to other groups of the Primates. Some zoologists thought it was an aberrant sort of lemur, some took the view that it was really a lowly type of monkey, and yet others, on account of the combination of primitive and advanced anatomical characters that it displays, regarded it as neither, but an intermediate type that deserved to be placed in a separate zoological group of its own. It was also interesting because it is the sole survivor today of a rich assortment of extinct 'tarsioids' that extended their range over considerable areas of the Old World and the New World many millions of years ago. In fact, it is generally believed that the higher Primates—monkeys, apes, and man himself—had their original evolutionary origin in one or other of these different groups of early tarsioids. When I settled in London I gave several of my specimens of *Tarsius spectrum* to my friend Dr Woollard, and on the basis of this material he published an outstanding monograph on its anatomy. My own studies of the creature were concentrated on its brain, with particular reference to that part of the brain called the thalamus, a complicated mass of grey matter through which messages from sensory organs are relayed to the highest functional levels of the brain, the cerebral cortex. From these studies I came to the conclusion that those zoologists were right who placed the tarsier (and the extinct tarsioids) in a separate group intermediate between lemurs and monkeys. I made further comparative studies of the brains of insectivores and lemurs, studies of a purely descriptive kind, and it was these that led me on to investigate the functional connexions of different parts of the brain by experimental methods. In the nineteen-twenties very little was known of the connexions and functions of various parts of the thalamus in the brain, and it was to this theme that I next turned my attention. But I will defer mention of these neurological studies to a later chapter in which I give an account of my explorations of the brain by experimental investigations.

As I have already indicated, my teaching duties at Bart's and Thomas's were heavy because in those days there was a very inadequate staff to assist me. But I enjoyed these duties, particularly those of demonstrating in the practical work of the dissecting-room that brought me into close personal contact with my students. Such a personal relationship not only gave me the opportunity of helping them in the progress of their studies in topographical anatomy, it allowed me to know them well as individuals and, from time to time, to give them advice by talking over with them intimate personal problems, not related to anatomy at all, that might be troubling them. This was a most important facet of the responsibilities of a professor in the London Medical Schools for, unlike Oxford and Cambridge, they had no college tutors to whom they might go for fatherly guidance in their personal affairs. I also enjoyed giving lectures—all except the first one I was due to deliver but did not deliver. And here I shall recount an incident that may surprise the many hundreds of students and others to whom I lectured during my academic career, for I soon gained a fair reputation as a lecturer. The incident may also be of interest to those who, like me, find the ordeal of the first lecture rather overwhelming. The fact is that on my way by underground railway to the medical school where I was due to give my first lecture I suddenly panicked—I felt I simply could not face the serried rows of a hundred or more students in the amphitheatre of ascending benches. I went past the station where I should have alighted, and at a station further on telephoned to say that I was unwell—a perfectly true statement for I was certainly unwell in my mind. But at the next lecture that I was due to give I forced myself to meet the occasion by recalling to myself the quotation from *Macbeth*—'be bloody, bold and resolute'. Incidentally, on more than one occasion later when I had to give some special address that gave me a certain amount of apprehension I often braced myself for the ordeal by exhorting myself with this quotation, and I commend it to others who may from time to time experience diffidence about their ability to fulfil some new responsibility that may come their way. When I did give my first lecture I found to my satisfaction that after an initial few minutes of trepidation I suddenly began to feel a sense of exhilaration in my delivery. Thereafter I continued to enjoy giving lectures, though it is an interesting fact, that even in my routine teaching to medical students extending over some forty years, I hardly ever approached the lecture theatre without that curious sinking feeling in the pit of the stomach. Indeed, on the very few occasions when I did enter the lecture theatre in a neutral state of mind, the lecture always seemed to 'drag' uncomfortably—the right words would not present themselves, phrases got mixed up, and the trend of my delivery did not follow its proper sequence. I soon came to realize, therefore, that in order to give out the best of oneself in a lecture, or for that matter in an after-dinner speech, it really is necessary to approach it with that degree of preliminary nervousness which, so to speak, tones one up for the occasion by (in some manner) enhancing one's cerebral activity. It may even lead to a sort of effervescing fluency that gives surprise to the lecturer himself.

There are some who take the view that formal lectures in the medical curriculum are unnecessary because there are always good text-books available for the student to read. I think this view is mistaken. For one thing, there are some students who gain a better grasp of their subject by auditory memory than by visual memory. The main purpose of a lecture, also, is not merely to give a systematic repetition of details to be found in text-books, but rather to arouse and stimulate interest by focussing attention on salient points, to make exciting to the student what is exciting to the lecturer. Clearly, therefore, a lecturer is not likely to be a successful lecturer unless he himself finds excitement in the subject on which he lectures. When I was in London, attendance at lectures was compulsory for medical students. But this was an ill-advised system and I was glad to find when I later came to Oxford that attendance at lectures there was entirely optional; the students did not need to go to all the lectures if they derived no benefit from them.

I do not know whether the beneficial advantages of what I would call 'physiological' nervousness have ever been system-atically studied, but I am convinced that in those of active and agile mind who regularly experience such a condition it is a normal phenomenon, and even essential to the success of their work. There are those who appear to take the view that any apprehensiveness about future possibilities should always be avoided on the grounds that these possibilities may never eventuate. Live for the moment, they say, and give no thought to contingencies that may not present themselves. But this is the attitude of mind of the care-free (and therefore careless), and of the unforeseeing. Foresight is surely a desirable trait in so far as it gives consideration to eventualities that are not expected to occur but are not unlikely to do so. A mild restlessness of mind of this sort does at least prepare in advance for meeting contingencies that may arise, and it also widens the horizon of contemplative thought by directing attention to possible, and perhaps more effective, alternatives to a course of action that has already been formulated. I suppose it is true to say that, in general, candidates for an examination approach the latter with feelings of apprehensiveness. At any rate they ought to do so, for (with very few possible exceptions) the most successful candidates are those who do experience a preliminary nervousness. Not only does this spur them on to their utmost effort in their preparation for the examination, it conduces to a mental alertness—a mental agility—that is of essential importance if a candidate is to give full expression to all those faculties of which he is capable in confronting his examination test.

I know a man of academic distinction who for many years started his day's work with a slight apprehensive feeling of inquietude. Psychiatrists might call this an anxiety neurosis, but to my way of thinking it is a biologically normal state of mind for those who face a busy day of uncertainties. Animals in the wild are constantly on the alert for possible dangers that may otherwise take them unawares. We ourselves have perhaps inherited the same tendency from our past ancestry, and it is natural enough, therefore, that we should continue to share this common mammalian trait. I have yet to meet the man with a reputation for gay and scintillating after-dinner speeches who does not admit that his enjoyment of a dinner is to some extent marred by the prospect of the ordeal that he will later have to face. I know of an eminent surgeon who, before undertaking an operation of unusual complexity, was seized with a degree of apprehensiveness that manifested itself in palpitations and diarrhoea, but he always carried out the operation with superb technical skill and outstanding success. I have also heard of a well-known sprinter who came to realize that he could not give his best performance in a race unless this was preceded by a premonitory nervousness, and if this feeling of nervousness did not arise of itself, he would do his best to arouse it deliberately by contemplating possibilities of failure.

Of course, there is no sharp dividing line between physiological and pathological states of anxiety; the latter will drain away energy just when energy is needed. I have occasionally had students of high calibre under my care who developed such an intense state of anxiety before an approaching examination that they felt they were simply unable to face it at all. These young men were in not a few cases the sons of distinguished fathers, and they had become so imbued with the fixed idea that they had a reputation to maintain that they were quite unable to contemplate any possibility of failure. It seems probable that this idea must have been unconsciously inculcated in their mind from such an early age that it had come to form an integral part of their personality, a completely dominating and obsessional theme from which they were helpless to escape by their own efforts. They needed to be treated with sympathy and understanding, but also with firm frankness, and my sessions with them were sometimes of a rather lengthy psychotherapeutic nature. 'Who do you think you are?' was the line I took—'Not everyone can always succeed in an examination. Why should *you* consider yourself to be so marvellously brilliant that you must on no account fail? Come off that pedestal of a talented genius that you have built up for yourself and be as other men are. You will almost certainly pass your examination, but if by chance you do fail be ready to accept the situation and regard it not as indignity but as an unlucky mischance' and so on. In most cases this line of approach was successful. But not always, for I recollect one student who in my time consistently fled from the prospect of an examination though, for all I know, he may subsequently have overcome his resistance to this 'ordeal'. No doubt such a man needs treatment by an experienced psychiatrist.

The life of a scientist in a university is by no means confined to departmental administration, teaching and research. There are sundry faculty board meetings to attend, and a variety of committees. And I always looked forward to the periodical meetings of the scientific societies of which I was a member. The Anatomical Society used to meet once a quarter, at one or other of the medical schools in London or in provincial universities, and these gatherings provided an opportunity of meeting fellow anatomists from many medical schools and of discussing with them matters of mutual interest. The meetings were followed in the evening by a dinner where we were able to continue our discussions in an atmosphere of pleasant conviviality. I also attended the meetings of the Royal Anthropological Institute, but less frequently because many of the lectures there dealt with ethnographical subjects rather far removed from physical anthropology that was my own interest. The Institute had a fine library, but it was housed in an old building entirely inadequate for the importance of a society that had had a long history of scientific contributions to the study of mankind of the present and mankind of the past. But it was seriously lacking in funds, the more surprising in those days considering the obligations of our Government towards the native inhabitants of our colonial territories and the need to familiarize ourselves with the development of their primitive social organizations so that these could be adapted to the changing world. I had been elected to the Fellowship of the Institute at an early stage of my medical career, and I particularly remember a lecture given by a man called Charles Dawson who had just recently achieved world-wide fame as the 'discoverer' of Piltdown Man. He gave all the appearance of a genial and open-minded amateur archaeologist, and in his lecture he was concerned to demonstrate that the small, shaped flint pebbles called 'eoliths' that had been found on the Sussex Downs and elsewhere were not tools deliberately fabricated by prehistoric man (as some had supposed) but were the result of fractures produced by natural agencies. In this conclusion he was no doubt correct, but later evaluations of some of his other archaeological work did raise doubts about his competence and even his honesty.

The meetings of the Zoological Society in Regent's Park I attended very regularly, and I always enjoyed them because they were lively and stimulating meetings at which many diverse subjects of great interest to me were discussed. The secretary of the Society at that time was Sir Peter Chalmers Mitchell, a man of no great distinction in the field of academic zoology but with a reputation for his administrative ability and for his popularization of current scientific affairs in the lay press. To some he appeared rather cold and aloof in temperament, but he gave me much encouragement in my early zoological studies. It seemed to me that his reticent disposition was curiously reflected by the appearance of his office in Regent's Park for it was strangely furnished in a scheme of monotonous black—black curtains, black carpet and black upholstery. Yet in a company that was congenial to him he could be very vivacious in conversation and anecdote. I saw this side of him from time to time at the Savile Club where he commonly used to lunch and dine, and of which I became a member in my London years. I felt it an unusual privilege to belong to this club, for it had a well-deserved name for its distinguished personalities in many branches of the arts and sciences. Particularly do I remember making the acquaintance there of Sir Ray

Lankester, then in his declining years at the age of about eighty, for in my student days I was stimulated to a high pitch of intellectual excitement by his writings. And he was one of the last close links with Charles Darwin and Thomas Henry Huxley with whom he had been acquainted in his younger days. He was a grand old man with a massive head that must have enclosed a brain of unusual capacity, and he was certainly the most distinguished and versatile zoologist of his period. He died in 1929, and I was interested to read in one of his obituary notices that for him 'the dissection of an animal was not a matter of dull routine but a voyage of exploration in which new discoveries might be made'. This was precisely the feeling that I had myself experienced when I came to dissect some of the less well-known animals that I had collected in Borneo. The superintendent of the Zoological Gardens was a close friend of mine, Dr Geoffrey Vevers, who, like myself had graduated in medicine from St. Thomas's Hospital. Chalmers Mitchell was occupied with so many outside interests that it was Geoffrey Vevers who assumed the main responsibility for the care of the animals by his day-to-day supervision of their living conditions and their feeding, and the immediate supervision of the administrative personnel and the staff of 'keepers'. Indeed, it was largely due to him that the organization of the Zoo was carried out so efficiently and so smoothly, and made so attractive to visitors by the floral displays that he designed for the gardens as well as by the display of the animals in their well-kept houses and enclosures. I have thought that he did not receive full credit for all that he had done for the Zoo in his days as its Superintendent.

No doubt one of the attractions of meetings of the Zoological Society was the Zoological Club to which I was elected in 1924, a small and, as we used to pride ourselves in those days, a rather select zoological company. We dined together after the scientific meetings, and it gave me the opportunity of particularly close and friendly contact with eminent zoologists, anatomists, and medical and other authorities of the day who were concerned with zoological matters. And from time to time we entertained distinguished zoologists from abroad. It was on one of these occasions that I first met Dr Robert Broom from South Africa, whom I was to know more intimately later when I visited that country. He was a little, wizened man who, in spite of his years, always displayed an amazing vitality and energy. He was primarily noted for his discoveries of the ancient mammal-like reptiles that inhabited the Karoo region of South Africa about 250 million years ago, and some of which were undoubtedly ancestral to the true mammals that initially appeared about 150 million years ago. Subsequently he made some most remarkable discoveries of the 'ape-men' of South Africa (the australopithecines as they are called) which had a place in our own ancestry, that is to say, the ancestry of *Homo sapiens*.

There were other societies, some of them local medical school societies and some general organizations in whose activities I was interested. Of these the Geologists' Association I found particularly useful. My knowledge of geology had previously been derived from reading and from exploring geological formations on my own account. But the Geologists' Association used to arrange excursions on Saturdays to the neighbouring countryside, each conducted by a professional geologist who had made a special study of the region, and occasionally longer excursions further afield. It was in this way that I began to gain a more practical knowledge of the subject that came to be of considerable use to me for assessing the geological evidence of the antiquity of fossil remains of early man. And, besides all these interests, like other university scientists some of my time was taken up with the conduct of examinations in London, in provincial medical schools, or abroad, with attendances at congresses, with visits to scientific institutions on the Continent, with special lectures that I was invited to give at the Royal College of Surgeons and elsewhere, and with occasional holidays in France, Holland, Austria and Switzerland. I suppose most of us, having reached our span of three score years and ten, look back on our earlier activities and wonder how we managed to accomplish our routine professional duties and to accomplish so much more besides. But, of course, our minds were more agile in those days, and I know I was capable of working more rapidly then than I am able to do now. As a continuing and happy background to all my work while I was in London was my home life at Digswell with my wife and my growing children, and I realize now, far more than I perhaps did at the time, how much I owed to Freda for her domestic care and for the selfless inspiration that she always gave me in the diversities of my work, notably the preparation of lectures and in the writing of my first book to be published. Such incidental work often took up much of my week-ends at home, interspersed with some necessary gardening. But, in spite of these diversions, we had at all times a very happy companionship, particularly on our holidays alone together or with our children.

CHAPTER 4

AN EXCURSION INTO ANATOMICAL HISTORY

I N 1930 there occurred the four-hundredth anniversary of
the death of an early anatomist, Berengario of Carpi, who
for much of his life was Professor of Surgery at Bologna.
According to the late Dr Charles Singer, one of the most
distinguished authorities on the history of science, his first
anatomical treatise was the earliest that can properly be
described as having figures illustrating the text. The Osler
Club at St. Bartholomew's Hospital asked me to celebrate the
occasion by reading a paper on the life of Berengario, and this
led me to a fascinating exploration of the literature bearing on
this anatomist. It was my first, and only, really detailed research into medical history. It was subsequently published
in the *St. Thomas's Hospital Gazette* where it has since lain
more or less hidden all these years, for the *Gazette* has only a
limited circulation. It has therefore seemed appropriate to
reproduce it here, and I do so in large part as a tribute to the
memory of my friend Charles Singer to whom I was indebted
at the time for references to some of the relevant literature. I
also acknowledge with thanks the present editor of the *Gazette*
for permission to reprint this essay.

*   *   *   *   *   *

This is the story of Jacopo di Faustino Barigazzi (Berengarius
Carpensis), whose four-hundredth anniversary is being celebrated this year at Bologna.

Somewhere towards the end of the fifteenth century, probably between 1480 and 1490, in the small town of Carpi,

about nine miles from Modena in northern Italy, the noted Aldus Manutius, classical scholar and pioneer in the art of printing, undertook the education of the small sons of the widowed Princess Caterina of Carpi. With them also he taught another boy, Jacopo Barigazzi, the son of a surgeon of local fame, Faustino Barigazzi. There can be little doubt that this small class was a lively one, and, at least in the case of Jacopo, Manutius must have found some difficulty in his endeavours to inculcate an enthusiasm for classical scholarship. For Jacopo, although in later years he wrote some valuable books and edited others, never acquired anything like a polished style of writing in the Latin language, or even a style that was grammatically correct. In truth, his interests probably lay in other directions. From his earliest childhood his father had taken the trouble to give him instruction in his own art of surgery and perhaps had even allowed him on occasion to help him in his work. So that Jacopo had developed an enthusiasm for what is sometimes termed a modern in contrast to a classical education. Nevertheless, he held a very great respect for his master and, in later life, he was wont to pay frequent visits to the old man and was clearly very proud of the honour of being included among his friends. And, if Jacopo was disappointing as a classical scholar, he undoubtedly was infected by Manutius' enthusiasm for the acquirement and the spreading of knowledge.

As he grew up, Jacopo became especially friendly with one of his aristocratic fellow pupils, Albert Pio, who, likewise, was athirst for knowledge of things of nature. It seems, indeed, that they were both tremendously interested in natural history and especially in that branch of the subject which we now call physiology. This enthusiasm even led them to cut open dead pigs in order to study the internal organs and to see how they worked. At first they looked upon this as rather an amusing game, but it was not long before they began to realize it was something more, and that here was a means of acquiring knowledge of a very important and practical kind. Jacopo himself, from the experience which he had already gained under his father's tuition, recognized the fundamental importance which a knowledge of anatomy and physiology must have for the practising surgeon and physician, and perhaps they both heard rumours of the tentative advances in the science of anatomy which had been made by Mondino at Bologna and Zerbi at Pavia. It is certain, at any rate, that Albert Pio, when he came of age and attained to the position of Seigneur of Carpi, resolved to do all in his power to aid the advance of all branches of knowledge, including anatomy, and to that end he used to invite savants and searchers after truth to his palace and to provide them with all the facilities which they might require. It is said that he initiated public dissections with the idea of promoting general education, that pigs were used for this purpose, and that the actual task of carrying out the dissections was delegated to Jacopo Barigazzi. Jacopo must have owed not a little of his later success to his enthusiastic and energetic friend, Albert Pio, and, indeed, he himself was the first to admit it. It appears that Jacopo had by now fully made up his mind to follow in his father's footsteps, and he accordingly went to Bologna to study and finally took the degree of Doctor of Arts and Medicine. What he did then is somewhat uncertain. It seems that he returned to his native town and settled in practice there, and very likely with his father who was still alive. But one gathers he was not altogether successful. Perhaps his attention was not sufficiently monopolized by his clinical practice. Being essentially endowed with the spirit of research, he may have found the life of a general practitioner not very congenial, but more than this, he allowed himself to be drawn into political troubles which were beginning to loom up in his neighbourhood, There was a certain antagonism between Albert Pio, local Seigneur of Carpi, and the Duke of Ferrara (a town some miles eastwards), who was then Governor of Carpi, an antagonism which was resolved some twenty-five years later by the complete domination of Carpi by the Duke of Ferrara and the disappearance of Albert Pio's line. However the matter arose, there is documentary evidence which shows that, in the year 1500, Jacopo Barigazzi was officially charged with being concerned in various plots against the Duke of Ferrara, and as the result he was ordered to pay a fine of one hundred ducats, or, if he refused, to have his nose cut off. His father paid the fine for him. The incident caused him to leave Carpi and once more to go to his old University at Bologna. He probably felt safer at Bologna, and, besides, he now felt ready to devote himself entirely to his professional work and especially his old hobby, the study of anatomy, and to break altogether with his associations of the past few years that had led him into such trouble. Perhaps that was one of the reasons why he changed his name about this time. He abandoned his family surname of Barigazzi and called himself Jacopus Carpensis or Jacopo da Carpi. It is obvious enough of course, that he took his name from his native town, and Zerbi, the anatomist (who died in 1505), must have known this even though he made the acid suggestion that the name of Carpi was to be derived from the Latin *carpere*, meaning to steal. But then Jacopo had evidently been at loggerheads with this predecessor of his, for he criticizes him with undue bitterness in the works which he published later.

Not only must Jacopo have been a man of brilliant intellect, but he must have impressed the authorities at Bologna very strongly with his ability and with researches which he had been engaged in, for, two years later, in 1502, he was appointed lecturer on surgery at the University. His election evidently proved a success from every point of view, for he held the Chair up to the year 1527. We have evidence, also, that his continuous and excellent service to the University was recognized by granting him an increase of salary in October 1507, December

1509, and lastly in April 1525. Moreover, he soon established himself as a man of merit in the city, for, in 1506, the freedom of the city of Bologna was conferred on him by Pope Julius II. From Jacopo's own point of view, the outlook must have been a very bright one in these early years of his appointment at Bologna University. He was in a position to prosecute his investigations in surgery and anatomy without interruption, and he could look forward to the many years of prosperity which were to come. He settled down to his studies, collecting for himself a library of such celebrated works as Avicenna, Albucasis, Cornelius Celsus, Guido, Theodoric, Lanfranc, etc., a library which assumed sufficient importance to receive special mention in the will which he made many years later. It is evident enough that he made good use of his library, and he was especially familiar with the writings of Celsus. He derived very considerable inspiration from the work of his predecessor, Mondino, whose *Anatomia* had been published some twenty years previously at Pavia, and though he found occasion later to criticize some of Mondino's observations, he always did so with the greatest feelings of respect for the famous anatomist. But though Jacopo was undoubtedly well acquainted with the authorities whose works were available in his time, one of his most outstanding characteristics was his critical faculty and his tendency to rely more on his personal observations and less on the written statements of his predecessors. That he did not altogether escape the influences of traditional anatomy is not surprising, considering the times in which he lived, but this in no way detracts from his fame as an original investigator of singular importance. His writings provide abundant evidence that he was an assiduous dissector, and he laid considerable stress on his advice that anatomy cannot be learnt by reading and listening to lectures but only by seeing and touching the actual body. According to his own statements, his school of anatomy at Bologna attracted large numbers of students, and it seems that his dissections were carried out in considerable detail. Whereas before him the public dissections consisted of little more than opening the body and revealing the internal organs *in situ*, Jacopo took the trouble to dissect in the true sense of the word and to separate the organs and tissues one from another so as to study their relations in an intimate fashion. His practical mind is shown by his discussion of the best kinds of body on which to study anatomy, and his assiduity by his remark that he often dissected numbers of bodies in order to settle some disputed or uncertain point. No doubt his dissections would be considered very imperfect in comparison with those which were made by his successors, Fallopius, Eustachius, Vesalius and others, but they marked a real step in the progress of anatomical study. Jacopo states that he dissected more than a hundred bodies. Even if this is an exaggeration, it seems certain that he did dissect a large number, and this may appear surprising in view of the general belief that the popular and religious prejudice against the mutilation of the dead body in those times made it extremely difficult for anatomists to obtain subjects for their dissections, and even forced them to carry out their dissections in secret. But this is by no means an accurate representation of the prevailing conditions. No doubt there were difficulties, and anatomists had to face a measure of antagonism from some of the officials of the Church. The notorious Bull, *De Sepulturis*, of Pope Boniface VIII in 1300, prohibiting the dismemberment of the human body and the boiling of human bones, was clearly directed against certain practices indulged in by the Crusaders, and there is no evidence that the Popes themselves ever endeavoured officially to suppress dissection. On the other hand, it is certain that the edict led to misunderstandings and misinterpretations by the Church. Mondino, in his work *De Anatomia Auris*, wrote that certain bones could only be properly recognized after boiling, but that he himself did not prepare them thus as he was fearful of committing a sin. Even Jacopo was aware of this ban, for he refers to this remark of Mondino and, indeed, says of him that he did not always offer resistance to this sin and, in spite of it, did sometimes boil human bones. Perhaps, also, this is why Jacopo advised that the best way to study osteology was to pay a visit to the local cemetery.

As a matter of fact, he may well have experienced difficulties in his relations with the lesser dignitaries of the Church, for there is a record of a letter sent to the Bishop of Tortona, Governor of Bologna, by Cardinal Bembo, in which the latter makes the unkind remark that Jacopo was a man who did not feel it wrong to tell lies about other people if by so doing he brought credit to himself. But it is clear that Jacopo found great favour with the Popes themselves, which would hardly have been the case if they had objected to his anatomical researches. It has been mentioned above that Pope Julius II honoured him by conferring on him the citizenship of Bologna. Cellini records that when Jacopo went on a visit to Rome the 'Pope would fain have had him in his service, but he replied that he would not take service with anybody in the world and that those who had need of him might come and seek him out'. This illustrates well enough the attitudes of the Pope to the anatomist even though the latter part of the quotation, if it is true, may indicate that Jacopo was not always a man of tact. There are a few more points which show that the Popes and Jacopo were on terms of friendliness or even of mutual respect. Pope Leo X, for example, arranged that one of his own relations, Alessandro Soderini, should undergo treatment by Jacopo. His successor, Clement VII, on another occasion got him to go to Piacenza in order to render surgical aid to one Giovanni delle Bande Nere, who had been wounded at Pavia. Lastly, the famous 'Commentary' of Jacopo was dedicated to Pope Julius II and shows on the frontispiece the emblem of Leo X.

In the year 1518 Jacopo published a treatise on fractures of the skull, entitled *De Cranii Fractura Tractatus*. This was not a very noteworthy piece of work. It is lacking in elegance and method, and the author rather slavishly follows the methods of Arabian medicine. But it is interesting because here Jacopo first uses the name Berengario by which he is usually known at the present day. Why he adopted this name is not known. There is a record in a papal Breve that he married a lady of a family of some standing, and it may be that he assumed her family name. In the *Tractatus* there are some verses in praise of the author written by one Bernadino Berengario, and this is evidence that there did exist a family of this name in Bologna. Possibly Jacopo had received assistance from this family and expressed his gratitude by taking their name. In the years 1521 and 1522 Berengario (as we may now call him) published two anatomical works. The first was a commentary on Mondino's Anatomy and was entitled *Commentaria, cum amplissimis additionibus, super Anatomia Mundini, cum textu ejus in pristinum nitorem redacto*. As the title indicates, this commentary is something more than a revised edition of Mondino's work, and the author has not hesitated to make corrections and add new information in a manner which bears witness to his powers as an original observer.

The second book was called *Isagogae breves perlucidae et uberrimae in anatomiam corporis humani, ad suorum scholasticorum preces in lucem editae, cum aliquot figuris anatomicis*. This book, which was dedicated to his old friend and fellow-pupil, Albert Pio of Carpi, contains a record of the author's personal observations, with many directions to the student for the dissection of the human body. It may well be regarded as the first practical anatomy text-book to be printed.[1]

---

[1] It is to be noted, in parenthesis, that a book published in London in 1664, under the title *A Description of the Body of Man, being a Practical Anatomy*, was commonly supposed to be a translation of the *Isagogae*, but this has been pointed out to be erroneous.

Both these books are illustrated. Indeed, they are the first text-books of anatomy to be illustrated by text figures, of which there are nineteen in the 'Commentary' and twenty-two in the *Isagogae*. It is well recognized that these figures occupy a very important place in the history of anatomical illustration. It has been supposed that they were actually engraved by the artist and wood-engraver, Hugo of Carpi, and they display a vigour of style and an artistic excellence which stand in strong contrast with the traditional anatomical schemata of those times. Representations of the human body, in various stages of dissection, are shown in life-like poses, displaying their muscles, their bones, and their entrails, in heroic attitudes in the midst of classical scenery in a style which clearly foreshadows (albeit to a limited degree) the superb illustrations published in later years by Vesalius. The figures do not, in themselves, disclose much progress in anatomical knowledge, but they herald the opening of a new phase in the production of anatomical treatises. They serve in part to fill in the gap between the anatomy of ancient tradition and the anatomy of Vesalius, and to indicate that the progress of anatomical science has, like Nature, not proceeded *per saltum*. Dr Singer, indeed, has pointed out some striking and suggestive resemblances to be found between certain illustrations from the works of Berengario and Vesalius, which would appear to indicate a close relationship between the two. Berengario may rightly be claimed a pioneer in many points of descriptive anatomy. He was the first to figure and describe the vesiculae seminales, to describe the caecal appendix, the hepatic circulation, the valvulae conniventes, and the sphenoidal air sinus; to show that the human uterus is not bicornuate as in other mammals and that the rete mirabile at the base of the brain is non-existent in man; to describe the arytenoids as separate cartilages and to give a clear account of the thymus; to perceive the sexual differences in the proportions of the thorax and pelvis; and, further, he gave more precise details than were hitherto available on many parts of human anatomy, and especially in regard to the structure of the larynx, kidneys, spinal cord, and brain.

These two treatises do not confine themselves entirely to anatomy. The author, for instance, allows himself to dwell on pathological curiosities, such as unusually early pregnancy, abnormally late menstruation, and cases of superfoetation, and, in the 'Commentary,' he relates an interesting case in which he removed a prolapsed uterus and effected a cure.

In addition to his anatomical work at Bologna, Berengario led a busy life as a surgeon, and his name today is especially associated with the treatment of syphilis which was then very prevalent in Europe. There is no doubt that he made a considerable reputation for himself in his methods of treatment, and it is interesting to read what Benvenuto Cellini has to tell about him. In Section XXVIII of the first book of his autobiography, Cellini says: 'There arrived in Rome a surgeon of the highest renown, who was called Maestro Giacomo da Carpi. This able man, in the course of his other practice, undertook the most desperate cases of the so-called French disease. In Rome this kind of illness is very partial to priests, and especially to the richest of them. When, therefore, Maestro Giacomo had made his talents known, he professed to work miracles in the treatment of such cases by means of certain fumigations; but he undertook a cure only after stipulating for his fees, which he reckoned not by tens, but by hundreds of crowns. . . . He was a man of much learning, and used to discourse wonderfully about medicine. . . . He was a person of great sagacity, and did wisely to get out of Rome; for not many months afterwards, all the patients he had to treat grew so ill that they were a hundred times worse off than before he came. He would certainly have been murdered if he had stopped.' And again in the second book, Section VIII, Cellini refers to 'that charlatan Maestro Jacopo, the surgeon from

Carpi. He came to Rome and spent six months there, during which he bedaubed some scores of noblemen and unfortunate gentlefolk with his dirty salves, extracting many thousands of ducats from their pockets ... and at the present moment in Rome all the miserable people who used his ointment are crippled and in a deplorable state of health.'

Those who have made their acquaintance with Cellini through the medium of his autobiography will readily admit that the disparaging references to Berengario may be discounted, interesting though they may be as the personal opinion of a great man. On the other hand, the complimentary remarks, may, by their very contrast, be accepted at their face value. That the great surgeon amassed a considerable fortune from his practice seems true enough, though the statement (attributed to Fallopius and to be seen in some of the posthumous editions of his book *De Morbo Gallico*) to the effect that Berengario, when he died, left a legacy of 50,000 crowns, besides a great quantity of plate, to the Duke of Ferrara, is certainly false. But, as his will shows, he left enough to build a College for Students of Medicine and to maintain there two or more Carpi scholars, in the event of his principal heir predeceasing him.

It has been commonly stated that Berengario was the first to treat syphilis by mercurial inunction, but the evidence is against this. Mercurial ointments had been used long before by the Arabians for leprosy and skin affections, and the same treatment seems to have had quite a widespread application with regard to syphilis as soon as this disease became rampant in Europe. But it is important to note that very diverse opinions were held as to the propriety of this method of treatment, and the latter formed the subject of some bitter controversies among the medical fraternity. Thus, Torella, physician to Pope Alexander VI, at the end of the fifteenth century, vigorously condemns mercurial inunction in the treatment of syphilis. He describes three forms of mercurial ointment, but says of them (quoting Freind) that 'they all destroy'd an infinite number of people, who in this case did not die but were downright kill'd: and these bold Empiricks must give an account, if not in this, in the next World of their practice, and be drown'd in the pit of repentance'. The adverse criticism of medical men, and the popular prejudice against mercurial inunction as indicated by Cellini's remarks, undoubtedly receives some justification from the fact that the mercury was supposed to cure by fluxing, producing salivation, and the poisons of the disease were believed to be eliminated in the outpouring of saliva. In other words, the inunction was pushed until toxic effects were produced. It is evident, therefore, that in pursuing the method of treating syphilis by mercurial inunctions, Berengario must have had to face considerable opposition from various sources. Perhaps his success was due to the fact that he recognized the significance of the toxic symptoms and was careful not to carry the treatment too far. But of this we know nothing. Attention may be called to the commonly repeated statement that Berengario treated Cellini for syphilis. So far as I know, there is no evidence for this. If one may judge from his remarks on Berengario as a syphilologist, Cellini would hardly have submitted himself to his treatment, and although in the second book of his autobiography he gives an account of his own attack of syphilis, he nowhere mentions Berengario in this connexion.

Berengario's long tenure of office at Bologna University, together with his great reputation as a practising surgeon, is sufficient evidence of a busy and prosperous career. As the years went by, he no doubt felt ready to lead a quieter life and devote more time to leisure occupations in which he had developed an interest. In July 1524 he bought a house in Bologna from one Gerolamo Ercolani, the Evangelist. This was evidently no mean estate, for with the house were a yard, stable, well, garden, and other appurtenances. Berengario was especially attracted by the garden, for in the following year he applied for and obtained permission to build a passage over the main road in order to link up his house with the garden and so allow free and ready access from one to the other. But if the garden was one of his interests, his collection of antiques and works of art must have provided him with the greatest joy. Many of these he no doubt acquired in the course of his professional work in lieu of monetary fees, as, for instance, Raphael's painting of John the Baptist, which is now to be seen in the Tribune at Florence, and which he obtained for services which he rendered to Cardinal Colonna. That he was a real connoisseur is clear enough from the remarks of Cellini, a man who was not ready to praise the artistic sense of other men unless he really admired it. Incidentally, Cellini records an amusing story which would seem to show that Berengario was not above passing off modern works of art as antiques to his friends. This is Cellini's story: 'He [Berengario] was a great connoisseur in the arts of design. Chancing to pass one day before my shop, he saw a lot of drawings which I had laid upon the counter, and among these were several designs for little vases in a capricious style, which I had sketched for my amusement. These vases were in quite a different fashion from any which had been seen up to that date. He was anxious that I should finish one or two of them in silver; and this I did with the fullest satisfaction, seeing they exactly suited my fancy. The clever surgeon paid me very well; and yet the honour which the vases brought me was worth a hundred times as much; for the best craftsmen in the goldsmith's trade declared they had never seen anything more beautiful or better executed. No sooner had I finished them than he showed them to the Pope; and the next day following he betook himself away from Rome. . . . He showed my little vases to several persons of quality; amongst others, to the most excellent Duke of Ferrara, and pretended that he had got them from a great lord in Rome, by telling this noblemen that if he wanted to be cured, he must give him those two vases; and that the lord had answered that they were antique, and besought him to ask for anything else which it might be convenient for him to give, provided only he would leave him those; but, according to his own account, Maestro Giacomo made as though he would not undertake the cure, and so he got them.'

It may have been that Berengario had intended to settle finally in Bologna, where he had spent such an active life. But, in 1529, he left Bologna and returned to Carpi, and is said to have entered the service of the Duke of Ferrara, Alfonso I, whose father he had been accused of plotting against in 1500. It would be interesting to know why he left Bologna. Nothing would seem more natural, one imagines, than that he should wish, after working for a quarter of a century in Bologna, to return once more to the town of his birth and of his family. There would, indeed, be little need to look for other reasons if it were not for the fact that, only a few years previously, Berengario had bought for himself a house and estate in Bologna, and had gone to the trouble and expense of building a bridge over the main road between the house and the garden. Perhaps it was failing health, together with the death of his only daughter, Faustina, in 1528, which decided his retirement to Carpi. His health had certainly not always been good, for we have a record showing that in 1521 he was granted sick leave on full salary. It may also have been such a circumstance which led him to make his will in 1528. Again, it may be that he wished to give personal aid to his relatives and fellow townsmen of Carpi in the frightful plague epidemic which raged there during the years 1527, 1528 and 1529, and which is reputed to have struck down half the inhabitants of the town. Whatever may have been his real reason for leaving Bologna, Berengario would without doubt have been not a little surprised if he could have anticipated the motives which were to be imputed to him by later generations. It was said that he had incurred the enmity of the Church, and fled in exile to Carpi (as though, indeed, he would have been any safer in Carpi than he was in Bologna). It was said he had to flee because he spoke in too ribald a fashion in public about his work of dissection; because he was too free in his conversation on certain matters which were regarded as obscene, such as the functions of the genital organs; and, again, because he had led a life of profligacy which ultimately got him into trouble. Worst of all was the story that, out of a personal hatred for the Spanish race in general, he had got hold of two Spaniards who were suffering from syphilis and dissected them alive, and as the result of this foul act, he had to escape the Inquisition. There is no evidence that any of these tales bears any relation to the truth. The accusation of vivisection, a common enough form of scandalmongering in those days where anatomists were concerned, is found in the posthumous editions of Fallopius' treatise, *De Morbo Gallico*, published at Padua in 1564 and 1566. It is not found, however, in the Venetian edition published in 1606, and it is this latter edition which authorities consider to be the most authentic reproduction of Fallopius' own work. Nor is there any reason to suppose that the reference of Boerhaave and Albino (in the introduction to Vesalius' *Opera Omnia*, 1725) to Berengario as 'verus Italorum Herophilus' contains an unpleasant imputation, or that it is anything more than a laudatory phrase. Berengario himself had declaimed against Erasistratus and Herophilus for their supposed vivisection experiments on the human body. He little realized that a similar false charge would be made against himself after his death.

There is perhaps an unfortunate tendency for stories of this kind, once they have been promulgated, to persist and cling with great tenacity to the history of the individuals about whom they were related, because they arrest attention by their very bizarre nature. There is all the more reason, therefore, to scrutinize them carefully and test them with collateral evidence. Certainly, in the case of Berengario, not one of these disparaging stories resists the test of scrutiny. More than that, they stand in direct opposition to the character of the anatomist as displayed by his career up to 1529.

The last piece of work which Berengario did before retiring to Carpi was to edit the anatomical works of Galen, and he dedicated this edition in 1529 to Cardinal Gonzaga.

When Berengario left Bologna finally, he must have been an old man, as age was counted in those days. Many of his relations had died, and he had no children of his own to survive him. His daughter, Faustina, had died, leaving him two grand-daughters, Faustina and Laura. Two of his sisters, Barbara and Thadea, the latter a widow, still lived. A third sister, Johanna, had died and left a son Gaspar. This nephew of his, Gaspar, was planning to follow in his uncle's footsteps and to be a doctor, and to him Berengario bequeathed in his will his medical books and his surgical instruments. Berengario's brother, John Andreas, was also dead, leaving a daughter, Ursulina, and a son, Damianum. Damianum was the principal beneficiary under Berengario's will of 28 March 1528, and to him was left everything with the exception of the legacy to Gaspar mentioned above, of a few articles of clothing to Barbara and Thadea, of a small sum of money to Ursulina, and of a thousand ducats to his granddaughters.

Berengario died on 24 November 1530, and he was buried in the Church of St. Francesco at Ferrara.

No better epitaph could well have been written to this distinguished man than the description of him by his successor Fallopius (*Opera Omnia*, 1606): 'Primus quoque omni dubio fuit anatomicae artis, quam Vesalius postea perfecit, restaurator.'

BIBLIOGRAPHY

Bembo, P. (1743). *Lettere*. Verona.

Berengario (1518). *De Cranii fractura*.

— (1521). *Commentaria super Anatomia Mundini*.

— (1522). *Isagogae*.

Choulant (1917). *History and Bibliography of Anatomic Illustration*.

Fallopius (1564). *De Morbo Gallico*.

— (1606). *Opera Omnia*.

Freind, J. (1727). *The History of Physic from the time of Galen to the beginning of the Sixteenth Century*.

Haesar, H. (1881). *Lehrbuch der Geschichte der Medizin*.

Hartwell, E. M. (1882). The study of human anatomy. *Johns Hopkins University Studies*.

Jourdan, A. J. L. (1895). *Biographie Médicale*, Vol. II.

Martinotti, G. (1923). *L'Insegnamento dell' Anatomia in Bologna*.

— (1923). *Il Testamento di Jacopo Barigazzi*.

Modestino del Gaizo (1893). *Dell' Azione dei Papi sul Progresso dell' Anatomia*.

Passavant (1839). *Rafael*, **1**, 303.

Portal, M. (1770). *Histoire de l'Anatomie et de la Chirurgerie*.

Puschmann (1891). *History of Medical Education*.

Rijnberg, G. van (1918). *Le Dessin Anatomique avant Vésale et de son Temps*.

Singer, C. (1925). *The evolution of Anatomy*.

Symonds, J. A. (1887). *The Life of Benvenuto Cellini*.

Vesalius (1725). *Opera Omnia* (prefaced by Boerhaave and Albino).

Walsh, J. J. (1911). *The Popes and Science*.

CHAPTER 5

A FLEETING VISIT TO RUSSIA IN 1931

IT was while I w s working in London that, in 1931, arrange-ments were made for a party of scientists and medical men and women to visit Soviet Russia on a tour of inspection of scientific institutions, hospitals and clinics, and at the same time to visit various places of more popular interest. I was glad to join this party because at that time I regarded the U.S.S.R. as a great experiment in social organization, possibly destined, as it seemed to me, to react strongly on the more conservative social organizations of other countries. Also, reports in the press on the progress of the Russian experiment were so varied, and often diametrically opposed to each other, that I wanted to see for myself what the real state of affairs might be. Naturally, like many others, I could not visualize how rapidly the new cultural system of the Soviets would eventually develop, though even then I was impressed with their emphasis on the need of great expansions in scientific research. But I was led to comment on the 'unmethodical mentality' of the average Russian worker and to surmise that this was really not a racial characteristic but rather the legacy of a prolonged cultural stagnation. In this I have proved to be correct, for the amazing technical efficiency of the Russian scientists today commands the respect of all scientists the world over. It is well to recognize this remarkable and rapid progress in technological achievement, for no-one can longer be in doubt that the Chinese are at least equally capable of similar spectacular developments in spite of their apparent cultural stagnation over the years gone by. One of the most outstanding scientists that I met in Russia was Professor Vavilov at the Academy of Agriculture in

Leningrad, a gentle and courteous man who spoke English fluently and had an international reputation for his studies of plant genetics. It was sad to learn later that, according to some reports, he had been 'liquidated' (in the phrase common at that time) and replaced by the notorious charlatan Lysenko who opposed all ideas of modern genetics on political as well as pseudo-scientific grounds. But it is some solace to know that 'Lysenkoism' has now been buried in the past with the complete vindication of all that Vavilov stood for in his own field of work.

I wrote a short account of my visit to Russia in the *St. Thomas's Hospital Gazette*, and I think it may be of some interest for readers to note my impressions of that country over thirty years ago. And so here they are.

*   *   *   *   *   *

It is estimated that between ten and twenty thousand tourists will visit the Union of Socialist Soviet Republics this year on sight-seeing tours. There can be no suggestion, therefore, that such a visit is in any way unique today. But only a trivial proportion of these tourists are of British origin, and this perhaps accounts for the fact that there is less general knowledge of modern Russia and the changes which are taking place there in England than in many other countries. Before leaving for Russia, indeed, one is apt to be regarded by friends and relatives as almost a pioneer who requires to be warned against undue rashness and to be accorded sympathy for the hard times which he is setting forth to endure.

The visit with which this short (and rather rambling) report deals was made by a party of scientists organized for the purpose of inspecting scientific and medical institutions in the U.S.S.R., and this special objective provides a further excuse for giving some account of it to readers of this *Gazette*. Naturally, no attempt is made here to give a systematic or exhaustive description of any aspect of life and progress in Russia and its relations to modern social and political problems. The author is no profound student of the philosophy of Marx and Engels, he does not profess an intimate knowledge of the history and problems of Communism, he has no previous acquaintance with Russia, and he is completely ignorant of the Russian language. He is not in a position, therefore, to do more than note some of his personal observations and experiences and to record his impressions uncoloured as far as is humanly possible by emotional bias. It will be apparent that a limited visit of eighteen days in a foreign country with almost complete dependence on interpreters can only allow of the most super-ficial study. When that country is Russia, which—so far, at least, as its social-political system is concerned—must by its very nature be in direct antagonism to every other country in Europe, the difficulties in the way of a visitor establishing any intimate contact with the native population are very much greater.

Let me first give a brief account of the purely personal side of our tour. We set sail in a Soviet steamer, the ss. *Rudzutak*, of some 3,000 tons, starting at London Bridge. This boat took us all the way to Leningrad, leaving London on 18 July and arriving on 24 July, having spent one day *en route* at Hamburg. The boat, which accommodated more than a hundred passengers as well as cargo, was very comfortable. Cabin accommodation was up to date and clean, and the food was both plentiful and appetizing. In general, there was little to indicate that the boat was owned and run under the direction of the Bolshevists rather than a private company. A certain lack of the spickness and spanness of the average British steamship might easily be paralleled in others of foreign origin. The appearance of one or two female deck hands with scarlet headkerchiefs was pictures-que rather than obtrusively striking, and the outward and

visible signs of smart discipline among members of the crew
are noted to be absent if deliberately sought for. Even so, there
seemed to be no lack of real discipline on duty. The ship's
routine day by day proceeded evenly and with little event of any
outstanding interest. We were given concerts and a cinema
entertainment by the crew, the latter consisting entirely of
propaganda films illustrating the progress of the Five Years'
Plan, especially that part which deals with the collectivization
of farms. The crew have cabin accommodation which, as far
as we could see, was precisely similar to that provided for the
passengers, and the captain was provided with a comfortable
two-room suite for his personal use. Without exception all the
Russians with whom we came into direct contact were of the
most friendly disposition and seemed to be all eagerness to
discuss their own problems of social reconstruction and to
learn about conditions in our own country. We never detected
any suggestion of a feeling of personal suspicion or animosity
such as might perhaps have been anticipated. On the boat we
were freely welcomed in the crew's quarters and we were
introduced here to our first acquaintance with a Lenin's
Corner. Every institution, community, or working unit in
Russia has its Lenin's Corner, a room or part of a room set
aside for the use of the workers, for recreation, study, meetings
and discussions of political and social matters. A prominent
feature is the bust of Lenin supported with decorations of red
bunting, and the walls abound with propaganda posters and
revolutionary slogans. On a notice board is posted the news
day by day, and here also complaints and suggestions may be
put up by any working member for consideration.

In Russia we had comfortable hotel accommodation. Indeed,
on occasion it might be called luxurious. At the October Hotel
in Leningrad, for example, I occupied a spacious room
provided with a telephone and with private bathroom
attached. In parenthesis, the telephones in Russia seem

extraordinarily unreliable, and with the aid of interpreters we had a good many struggles to get through to people whom we wished to meet. The food in the hotels varied somewhat. It was always adequate though sometimes unappetizing. The meat was often coarse, and Russian eggs are usually distinctly unpalatable. The drinking water in most places (except Moscow) is chlorinated, and we were advised to rely rather on mineral waters because of the prevalence of typhoid. For the same reason many of us felt rather diffident in partaking of the salads provided. Russian diet is certainly not suitable for an irritable colon.

Travelling by train or river steamer we found quite comfortable so far as the accommodation was concerned. In the trains one travels 'hard' or 'soft', i.e. in carriages with unupholstered or upholstered seats, four to a compartment. We tried both. The latter method is as comfortable as a third-class sleeper on a British railway, and the former almost so, since mattresses were provided at night. In both cases we were supplied at night with clean blankets, pillows, sheets and pillowcases, and I personally always enjoyed restful nights in the train. The lack of anything in the nature of a restaurant car on a long train journey makes it necessary to provision oneself in advance, always taking into account the possibility of the train being delayed several hours. Between Leningrad and Moscow the trains run smoothly and to time. On the other hand, our train journey from Stalingrad to Moscow was dismally slow, the track was poor, and we started five hours late.

Russia during August may be uncomfortably hot, and tropical clothing is a boon. Two or three of us spent most of our days in Russia in khaki shirt and shorts, and it surprised me what interest this mode of attire attracted, especially as it is so commonly adopted by men in central European countries in hot weather. People would turn round in the street, stare and laugh. One of our guides commented on our comfortable and cool appearance, and when I asked him why he did not wear similar clothes himself, he replied that he would like to but that he hardly dared because his friends would think he had gone crazy. Evidently the modern Russian is not so freed from the limitations of convention as one might imagine.

With the heat, the flies were a persistent nuisance. To a light sleeper they are a real pest in the early hours of the morning, and they were responsible for almost the only point of criticism which we could find in the excellent hospitals in Moscow.

Our tour in Russia lasted eighteen days. Of these we spent four days in Leningrad, eight days in Moscow, one day in Stalingrad, and four days going down the Volga. There is nothing to recommend the river trip on the Volga from the scenic point of view. We did not even hear any Volga boatmen singing the Volga boat song. The country all along is extremely flat and featureless, and the river is so broad that it is difficult to gather much information from a scrutiny of the banks. Our objective on this part of the journey was Stalingrad, which is situated in southern Russia, close to the Caspian Sea. Here, with the development of gigantic tractor factories, an industrial town of considerable size has developed out of the comparatively small fortified town of Tsaritsin. Now, as to general impressions. The impressions of a tourist in Russia no doubt depend to a considerable extent on his preconceived ideas of the country as well as upon his emotional reactions towards the political aims of the Soviet Government. I have no doubt, therefore (indeed I know for certain), that the impressions gained by different members of our party varied considerably. As regards the first factor, it is essential to start off with some historical point of view whose perspective is in accordance with the facts. In the first place, it must be realized that in pre-war days the state of the country was such that 73 per cent of the population were totally illiterate and the infantile mortality in the first year of life in some rural districts reached the appalling total of 50 per cent. To anyone with imagination, these two facts alone are sufficient to give a pretty good idea of the stage of civilization to which the Russian nation had then attained. Add to this the fact that in 1917, after three years of the Great War, the most disastrous civil war ever known broke out in a series of revolutions which culminated in an unprecedented famine in 1921, and the visitor will be prepared not to see a country in an efficient state of running order like other European countries, but rather a country in the slow process of laborious recovery from a condition of utter chaos. He will then interpret inefficiency and dilapidation not necessarily as the direct result of a new political system which may be distasteful to him, but rather as the heritage of the unhappy years of the past. His attention will thus be more attracted by the evidence of growing efficiency and orderliness in contrast to the many evidences of inefficiency and lack of method which still remain.

Of the places which we visited, Moscow without doubt shows the greatest evidence of the progressive consolidation of an efficient social system. As one wanders through the busy streets of this town, one mingles with throngs of people with every appearance of contentment and physical well-being, adequately and (in the case of the women) even gaily dressed. It is true, of course, that the average Russian still lives on what we would call a restricted diet, and is rigidly rationed in regard to practically all the necessities of life, but I was interested to note that wherever I went the people appeared healthy enough. So far as the children are concerned, indeed, their general appearance of blooming health is really rather striking. We certainly did not see any signs of starvation in any part of Russia which we visited. One of our party on one occasion partook of a factory mid-day dinner with the workers, and, according to his report, the food was the best he had tasted during his stay in Russia. As we were at that time staying at the Grand Hotel in

Moscow, where the food would have satisfied any but the professed gourmet, this recommendation was to me especially significant. Beggars are often an indicator of the degree of poverty in large towns. I counted three beggars during a week's stay in Moscow, and I imagine this is worthy of remark in view of their notorious prevalence in pre-war days.

A tremendous activity is noticeable in connexion with the reconditioning of Moscow generally. The old cobbled streets are being pulled up and replaced by road surfaces of modern construction. Old and inconvenient buildings are everywhere being demolished and huge blocks of flats for workers' dwellings and government offices are springing up. We were told that during the present year it is hoped that about 7 per cent of the town buildings will be pulled down and replaced by modern housing accommodation, and that by the end of the year accommodation for another 180,000 workers will have been completed. Even the large Cathedral of the Redeemer, which with its domes of gold looks fine enough in the distance, but close at hand is seen to be an unattractive building, is about to be demolished to make place for a Palace of Labour.

The rapid growth of the population of Moscow is evidenced by the overcrowded state of the tramway and motor-bus services, and this, we learnt, is to be remedied by the construction of underground railways which will commence next year. There is a considerable amount of traffic in the centre of Moscow, and here automatic light signals are used for traffic control. In its spare time, the populace of Moscow seems to know how to enjoy itself. We visited Stanislavsky's Opera House one evening to see the opera *Eugene Onegin* of Pushkin and Tchaikowski, and the house was filled to the last seat with a highly appreciative working men's audience. On another evening some of us went to the large Park of Culture and Rest, on the south bank of the Moskva. Here there are well laid out grounds with ornamental flower-beds, grass plots for games and athletics of all sorts, open-air concert platforms, exhibitions demonstrating the progressive industrialization of Russia and the progress of the Five Years' Plan, educational pavilions with demonstrations of agricultural, technical and biological scientific principles, cinemas, circuses, roundabouts, giant-wheels, community singing (with revolutionary songs, of course), community dancing, etc. The park was obviously very well attended and the crowds were remarkably orderly. As everywhere in Russia, full use is made here of the opportunity for the display of political propaganda, and at strategical points one comes across hoardings covered with large posters denouncing the machinations of foreign capitalists in no uncertain terms. A few of us joined in the community dancing, an instructive and even somewhat impressive experience, for it gave one an intimate and personal glimpse of the communal spirit which seems to be manifesting itself with such force in the Russian masses today. This community dancing takes place in a huge oval arena around which all the participants arrange themselves in a ring. We estimated that we altogether made up a dancing party of some 800 people. At one side is a covered platform with a band, and loudspeakers are placed at intervals over the ground. Before we start, the 'master of the ceremony' explains by means of the loudspeakers the details of the dance about to be played. These are perfectly simple. Perhaps a few trips forward, a pirouette with one's partner, a few simple side-steps, claps of the hand, a turn-about and tripping steps back. The different figures of the dance are demonstrated to us with the music by girls who are placed at intervals within the ring of dancers, and when we thoroughly understand the procedure the band starts in earnest and the whole 800 of us are off. A most exhilarating form of amusement that leaves us all breathless and eager for more. We were surprised how easy it is thus to secure a co-ordinated action of so many people in a community dance of this kind after such short instruction.

We also visited the large bathing establishment along the banks of the river Moskva and enjoyed our swim among throngs of seemingly happy workers. There must have been well over a thousand people of both sexes in full enjoyment of the swimming and diving facilities, or sun-bathing and playing tennis and other net games in their bathing slips. Most of them displayed a fine physique, and all of them were richly tanned with the sun. In Leningrad, as compared with Moscow, one receives a somewhat different general impression. Here there is still abundant evidence of the ravages of civil war. The main street, Prospect 25 October, which in pre-war times was a fashionable shopping centre, is in a very poor state of repair, and the fine buildings are badly in want of renovation. The street crowds have not that appearance of alertness and contented well-being that one notices in Moscow. Rather they seem to reflect the general drabness of their surroundings. On the other hand, the people are adequately clothed and they look fit enough physically.

On our way down the Volga we were able to spend a few hours in Samara and Saratow, and here the conditions of life appear less attractive. Climatically they are at a disadvantage, and the dusty streets on a windy and sweltering day are most unpleasant, as we ourselves experienced. These southern towns, also, bore to a much greater extent the brunt of the civil war and famine. It is not uncommon to see here unkempt individuals in very ragged clothing such as were not to be seen in Moscow and Leningrad.

Everywhere we went we were inevitably made aware of the immense amount of propaganda which is being carried on. Not only is one confronted with posters of great variety illustrating the progress of the Five Years' Plan and advertising the imminence of a world revolution, but one hears of shock brigades and agitating brigades who penetrate into all parts of the U.S.S.R., urging the people to complete their quota of the

CPE I

Five Years' Plan, teaching revolutionary songs and slogans, and generally doing all they can to raise them to the highest pitch of enthusiasm. On our way down the Volga we had the opportunity of hearing the methods of one of these agitating brigades, and they played their parts very well. In Leningrad we visited a cinema, and in the vestibule of the theatre there were exhibits of all kinds demonstrating the progress of industrialization in Soviet Russia, while in another part of the entrance hall a speaker was holding forth in enthusiastic tones to an audience of people waiting for the next performance on the successful prosecution of the Five Years' Plan. The film which we saw was a Russian 'talkie' entitled *The Way into Life*, and dealt in a very dramatic way with the methods which the Government have adopted to rescue the crowds of homeless waifs which used to infest the cities up till quite recently. Incidentally, we did not see any signs of these pariah children in any place which we visited. The Russians are expert propagandists, and for the moment, at any rate, they seem to be achieving their object. It remains to be seen whether, in the face of inevitable delays in the attempt at the final stabilization of the Soviet system, it will be possible to maintain the whole population on the crest of a wave of enthusiasm for a sufficiently long time. There is no doubt that the Russian masses are still living in very hard times and that they are still very strictly rationed for the necessities of life. They seem to be sticking it remarkably well so far, but many critics have raised the question as to whether human patience is sufficient to see them through. Probably in their case it is, for, to put it mildly, they are reluctant to return to pre-war conditions. Indeed, it has been said that any attempt to restore the old regime would bring about a revolution as bloody as the last.

In and around Moscow and Leningrad we saw plenty of evidence of military activities in the form of troops on the march, often singing revolutionary songs as they marched.

Whether this is the usual state of affairs or whether it is merely in association with the summer manoeuvres which are so conspicuous over most of Europe at this time of year, I am unable to say. If you make enquiries with reference to the extensive militarization which is going on in the U.S.S.R., you will be told that it is purely for protective purposes. If you were to suggest that this is unnecessary, you would be laughed at. The Russians are convinced disciples of Karl Marx, and they interpret the economic difficulties and financial crises in which most European countries are now involved as evidence of the imminent collapse of Capitalism which was prophesied by this philosopher half a century ago. Basing their arguments also on Marxian principles, they assert that the death struggles of Capitalism are certain to lead to a last desperate attempt to overcome the economic competition of Socialist Russia by force of arms, and they point to the evidences of military preparation in neighbouring states. Moreover, the Communists feel particularly vulnerable at this particular juncture when the accomplishment of their vast economic programme has still to be realized. If you enquire whether, in the event of a proletarian revolution in another country, the Soviet Union would use its army in an aggressive sense, your question would be met with an emphatic denial, for the Communists affirm that such a revolution would not lead to any final success unless the proletariat of the particular country involved is itself strong enough to gain the mastery without outside assistance.

During our stay in Russia we spent the greater part of our days visiting scientific and medical institutes. We also found time for sight-seeing of a more general nature, and besides visits to museums, art galleries and the old imperial palaces, we found time for a rapid survey of various aspects of social life under the Soviet socialist system, including visits to workers' flats, rest-homes, a prison, a registry office for marriage and divorce, a law-court, a prophylactic institute for women prostitutes, etc. I do not propose in this short account to deal with more than a very few aspects of life in Russia today as we saw it.

Let me mention a few specific points which occur to me and about which I have been asked since my return.

As regards religion. We looked into several churches in Leningrad and Moscow, and in some we came upon services in progress and, in some cases, with a crowded congregation. This will perhaps surprise some people who may have imagined that all priests have been ruthlessly exterminated. Of course the Soviet Government discourages religion and refuses to allow religious education in schools. But free permission is given for any church to continue in full activity so long as there is a congregation that can support it. Actually, in very many cases, it is impossible to do this, and the church is then taken over by the State for secular uses. This has happened, for instance, in the case of the Cathedral of St. Isaac in Leningrad. This huge and historical building sank into such a poor state of repair that it showed signs of becoming dangerous. It has been taken over by the Soviet Government and restored and, curiously enough, converted into an anti-God museum. We visited this museum. It consists largely of a series of exhibits demonstrating the progress of the Five Years' Plan, and the conditions of life of the workers in pre-war days, at the present day, and as they are expected to be in the near future. Another exhibit shows the various stages through which it is supposed that religion has evolved from primitive magic. There are numbers of photographs and life-size models showing the gorgeous vestments used by the priests on different ceremonial occasions, contrasting them with the poverty of the pre-war peasant. Other models illustrate the various 'freak' religions that have sprung up in Russia from time to time. Still further exhibits are designed to prove that the Russian Church was essentially a capitalist and counter-revolutionary institution. Thus there are reproductions of propaganda posters which were issued by the Church in the early days of the revolution showing the revolutionaries being struck down by fire from Heaven while the Tsar and his family stand protected by angels, while other pictures indicate how the Church amassed wealth by means of its candle factories, printing presses and other means. There is no attempt in this museum to ridicule religion by the sort of crude and ribald satire which one sees in some of the anti-clerical periodicals which were published on the Continent in other countries besides Russia. It is interesting to speculate what will be the ultimate result of this attempt to deprive a whole population of religion of any kind. One wonders whether a violent anti-God movement in one generation may not be succeeded by an anti-anti-God movement in the succeeding generation. This remains to be seen. The eagerness of the Communists to dispel the fog of religious superstition which has involved the ignorant Russian masses for so many centuries may perhaps be understood when it is realized that they are, for example, striving to instil some idea of scientific agricultural methods into the minds of a peasantry which hitherto has relied for good crops mainly upon due attention to the family ikons and sprinkling the ground with holy water. On the other hand, the total and final abolition of all religion and of the idea of God is a fundamental element in the philosophy of Communism. This is adequately expressed in the Marxian phrase which is today inscribed on the walls of the House of the Moscow Soviet at the north end of the Red Square, 'Religion is Opium for the People.'

In regard to the progressive industrialization of Russia, I am not in a position to say much from personal observation. There are plenty of figures available in official publications which indicate the advances which have been made in the last few years: 323 new factories were started into activity between 1927 and 1930, and it is proposed to complete and get going no fewer than 518 more new factories during the current year. We were taken round the famous tractor factories in Stalingrad which give some idea of the ambitious aims of the Five Years' Plan. There is no doubt that the Soviet Government is meeting with innumerable difficulties in the attempt to fulfil their industrial programme, and it is interesting to note that they quite freely admit this. Thus, in an account of the Stalingrad factory in the *Workers' News* published in Moscow on 1 August of this year it is stated that whereas it had been anticipated that by July the factory should have been producing ninety tractors a day, actually the output averaged only fifty-one. This is largely due to the tremendous amount of scrap material produced. Indeed it is said that, in many cases, more scrap parts are produced than good ones. Such a reason, of course, implies technical inefficiency of an unusual degree, and this without doubt represents the greatest obstacle which has to be overcome by the Soviet Government. The multiplication of factories is certainly an achievement of some magnitude, but obviously full advantage cannot be taken of these increased facilities for production on a large scale unless an adequately trained personnel is forthcoming. Attempts are being made to accelerate the education of skilled technicians of all kinds, but, unlike more concrete objectives, a five years' syllabus of education can hardly be compressed into three years without serious detriment. In the selection of candidates for such training, proletarians are usually given preference, and from the start the Soviets have poor material for their specialized educational work. I do not mean that the average Russian worker is dull and unintelligent, but his background of general education is necessarily limited and the lack of a broad intellectual culture is a serious handicap. The average Russian worker, again, is characterized by a slip-shod and unmethodical mentality. He has been a fatalist for so many centuries that it is almost as if he had forgotten how to work on his own initiative. Temperamentally he is rather irresponsible and lacks the power of organizing his own work satisfactorily. He takes little account of time and is rarely punctual, and, unless strictly supervised, he easily falls into slovenly habits. These traits remind one very forcibly of the lack of system and the poorly developed faculty for organization which seem so pronounced among certain Oriental peoples. Some would perhaps regard such temperamental characteristics as racial features. I imagine, however, that they are much more likely to be the result of a prolonged cultural stagnation. As I have indicated above, a tremendous campaign of propaganda is being carried on in order to rouse the Russian masses to a sense of their collective responsibilities. This campaign has been successful in creating a spirit of enthusiasm, but it cannot make up for a defective education. This is going to be a serious problem when the present older generation of scientific men has passed away. A great deal of the success and progress of scientific institutions in Russia today seems to be due to the efforts of men who have been trained in pre-war universities and who have had a generous education. When they have disappeared, will there be an adequate supply of sufficiently matured minds left to carry out the vast plans of industrialization and the development of technical and other sciences? At the moment there are considerable numbers of foreign technical experts, mainly American and German, in Russia, who are assisting in the organization and running of the new factories. What the standard of these experts is I cannot, of course, say but possibly in their own country they would not be regarded as men of any special ability. They do not always seem to work harmoniously with the Russians, for the complaint is made that, in the Stalingrad plant, for instance, one of the main shortcomings in the past has been the almost complete lack of contact, and in some cases even hostility, between the American and Soviet engineers.

We visited a number of medical institutions of various kinds during our stay in Moscow. There has been a considerable amount of reorganization, re-equipment and additional construction of hospitals and clinics since the revolution, and there seems no doubt that the city of Moscow is fairly well provided with medical facilities for its population of two million. One of the biggest hospitals is the Botkina General Hospital, where we spent one morning. We were conducted round by Professor Rosanoff, and it may be of interest to note that on entering the hospital we were all made to put on clean white overalls. We had a similar experience in visiting children's clinics. After being shown a small scale model of the hospital grounds and buildings and listening to a general account of the work of the hospital, we made a tour of the wards and various departments. The hospital holds 2,000 beds and is staffed by 10 resident doctors and about 150 visiting doctors. So far as we could see, the equipment was quite admirable, and especially was this noticeable in the departments of neurology, physiotherapy, hydrotherapy and electro-cardiography, where all the most recent types of apparatus from Germany were installed. The wards were comfortable and airy, and I was interested to see that besides the large wards there were quite a number of small wards for one or two patients that were used for special cases. The case sheets for each patient were astonishingly elaborate and must require a considerable amount of time for their completion. Incidentally, these case sheets from all the hospitals are eventually filed in a central bureau in Moscow, where they are available for statistical research on a big scale. The out-patients' departments were extensive and well arranged, and, as in all the clinics which we visited, the walls are covered with illustrated posters demonstrating hygienic methods of all kinds for education of the out-patients. We also saw the operating theatres, which were of up-to-date construction. On another day we went to a factory clinic, established in connexion with a factory with 11,500 operatives. Here there is accommodation for 200 in-patients in addition to well-equipped out-patient and special departments. Not only the workers, but also their families, are treated here, all free of cost. There are six of these clinics already in Moscow, and it is proposed eventually to establish sixteen altogether. We inspected also the Institute for Occupational Diseases, with about 200 beds as well as the out-patient clinics, and the Institute of Dietetics, with similar facilities for in-patients and out-patients, and laboratories for research. This institute is engaged in a comprehensive study of the optimum diet necessary for workers who are engaged in different kinds of work under varying conditions, and it provides the scientific basis upon which the numerous communal kitchens springing up all over Russia are controlled and directed. The Central Institute for the Protection of Mother and Child is an indication of the efforts which the Soviet Government is making for the provision of a healthy new generation. It represents a large ante-natal and post-natal clinic with wards and nurseries for the accommodation of babies who may require special care and nursing during the first few years of their life. Health propaganda is especially evident here, and there is quite a large museum of posters illustrating correct ante-natal preparations, the right and wrong way of looking after babies, the advantages to mothers and children of the new social system with its provision for women workers during pregnancy and after child-birth and its regulations governing the procedure of marriage and divorce, models of sanitation in houses and hygienic arrangement of living-rooms, exhibits of different appliances for the purpose of birth-control with their several advantages and disadvantages, life-like wax models illustrating the various disorders and diseases to which mothers and babies are liable, etc. On the outskirts of Moscow and Leningrad, also, there are numbers of children's homes for weakly or tuberculous children as well as crêches in which working mothers can leave their children for the day or for longer periods. I think we were all impressed with the good conditions under which these children were cared for as well as with the healthy and bonny appearance of the children themselves.

Abortion clinics are a peculiar feature of Soviet Russia. Some of us visited one of these clinics and were able to observe first-hand the technique used for procuring abortions. Usually a general anaesthetic is not used, and the gynaecological members of our party expressed the opinion that the operator, in using a sharp curette and applying it with considerable vigour, must almost certainly run the risk of a high percentage of complications. According to the verbal statement of the doctor, however, complications were very uncommon. It was said that 20,000 abortion operations were performed every year at this clinic alone. I tried to ascertain under what circumstances these abortions are produced, but it was not very easy to get a clear statement on the matter. My impression is that every pregnant woman up to the third month can theoretically demand an abortion if she wishes it. In actual practice, however, she is questioned as to her reasons for wanting it, and unless she can produce evidence of ill-health, economic distress, or some other adequate reason, she is dissuaded from undergoing the operation. It appears therefore that a good deal is left to the judgment of individual doctors as to the advisability of granting an application for an abortion. We were told that in Moscow altogether 70,000 abortions were induced annually. This, of course, is a large enough number in a population of two million.

I was interested to find out something about medical education in Soviet Russia. Unfortunately, during August medical schools are closed down for the vacation, and I was thus unable to study them in action. However, I had an interview with the director of the medical faculty of the First

Moscow State Medical Institute, from whom I learnt something of the educational methods.

The preliminary training before entering on a medical course consists either of a nine years' schooling (in schools which are approximately equivalent to secondary schools in this country) or a three years' course in a workers' faculty for those who are already trained in some other line of work. The number of vacancies at a medical school are advertised annually and applicants are chosen first from those of strictly proletarian origin and on the strength of their diplomas. Sixty per cent of the medical students in Moscow at the present time are women. This large proportion is due to the fact that men are attracted more by technical work, and there is, of course, a tremendous demand for skilled technicians just now. A medical student has four years' academic training, and after that he works as a clinical assistant for one year before he is entitled to a diploma of qualification. According to the last programme of the Council of People's Commissars, a school year consists of thirty decades. Each decade consists of two five-day periods. Thus the student spends approximately 300 days at work during the year. During the first year he devotes 306 hours to morphology (which includes topographical anatomy and the dissection of the cadaver, histology, and embryology), 264 hours to chemistry (organic, inorganic, physical and colloidal), and 174 hours of biology. Later in the curriculum there is a special course in medical physics for those who intend to specialize in physiotherapy. During the second year the student studies physiology, normal and pathological (326 hours), microbiology (144 hours), pharmacology and toxicology (120 hours), special hygiene (132 hours), morbid anatomy (60 hours), foreign languages, especially German (120 hours), and dialectical materialism (120 hours). This last subject appears rather odd in a medical syllabus. Broadly speaking, it involves a study of the philosophy of Marx and Engels in its relation to medical sciences and the relation of medicine to the Communist State. It has thus a political significance and serves to illustrate the fact that under the Soviet system of education every branch of work is given a political orientation. During the third and fourth years the student is engaged in clinical studies. Starting in the third year, each student selects some speciality and modifies his curriculum accordingly. The subjects in these courses include surgery, medicine, neurology, therapeutics, gynaecology and obstetrics, balneology, venereal diseases, physiotherapy, dermatology and stomatology.

During the first year the student also works as an ambulance man during the summer. Subsequently he acts as chief of the ambulance, and then during his third and fourth years he gains some practical experience as assistant to a practising physician.

There are no examinations in the medical curriculum. The professors, teachers, and the students themselves estimate the progress of each individual student throughout his career. Brigades of students are organized by the Students' Committee, and in each brigade a leader is appointed who is called a 'brigader'. If a student in a brigade is lagging behind his comrades in his work, the latter give him a helping hand. By means of social competition and the activities of shock brigades, it is claimed that the students are kept up to the mark and prevented from neglecting their work. At frequent intervals the brigades assemble together, and in the presence of the professor report on their work. The brigader reports the attendances of the members of his brigade and draws attention to any slackness or other defect. The brigades also join in 'academic battles' in which they put questions to each other on the work in which they are engaged, and the progress of each student is judged by the nature of the questions which he asks as well as by his answers. It is claimed that in practice these methods work quite satisfactorily. Attendances at lectures and classes are said to be remarkably regular and the students work keenly. Practically every student acquires his diploma at the end of his academic course. Students pay no fees, and all those requiring State scholarships for their maintenance are entitled to apply for them, and they are given such financial assistance as they may need. In addition to the medical schools, there are five post-graduate schools in Moscow.

This is a bald account of the general methods of medical education in Moscow. What the end result is, I cannot say. The fact that practically every student gets his diploma at the termination of the scheduled curriculum makes one feel that the standard required for the diploma cannot be very high. I would have liked to have interviewed students at the end of their second year and again immediately on qualification, and to have interrogated them on their work. Only by this means would it be possible to assess the value of the Russian medical education of today, and to effect a comparison with the knowledge acquired by the average English medical student at equivalent stages in his curriculum.

Perhaps no aspect of the modern social reconstruction of Russia is more remarkable than the tremendous scientific activity which is manifesting itself in all branches of science. Especially is this noticeable in the realm of industrial and agricultural research. Research laboratories are being multiplied throughout the Soviet Union at what seems to be an incredible rate, and it is claimed that during the current year there are 40,000 workers who are engaged exclusively in scientific research work. It is evident that all the forces of science are being mobilized to their fullest extent in order to advance the cause of Communism, and all scientific research is being directed with the precise object of assisting in the improvement and socialistic reconstruction of industry and agriculture in the U.S.S.R. We visited a number of institutes and laboratories, including the Lenin Academy of Agricultural Sciences in

Leningrad, Pavlov's famous Institute of Physiology, and the University of Moscow.

As far as we saw, the laboratories were well equipped and adequately staffed, and we understood that the scientific workers could always get what apparatus they required.

The Academy of Agriculture, presided over by Professor Vavilov, is an institution of vital importance to Russia. It consists of a large number of institutes such as the Institute of Plant Industry, of the Mechanization of Farming, of Plant Protection, of Agricultural Soil Science, of Drought Control, of Microbiology and Fermentation Processes, of the Electrification of Agriculture, of Animal Husbandry, etc. It took us the greater part of a day to see round the central offices of the Academy and the Institute of Plant-Breeding, spending only the briefest time in the various laboratories, plant-breeding grounds, testing stations, etc. Immense collections of cereals, etc., are stored here, which have been gathered in the course of expeditions which the Soviet Government has despatched to every quarter of the globe. Thus, for instance, the section for wheat is in possession of the largest collection of wheats in the world, containing more than 25,000 specimens from almost every country. The academy deals with the large-scale problems arising in connexion with the great development of agriculture in Russia, searching for the best type of crops for planting under the varying and often difficult climatic conditions of the country, investigating the question of mechanization of agriculture, and generally providing the scientific basis upon which the big collective farms are directed and controlled. At the recent International Congress of the History of Science and Technology, held in London, Vavilov gave a short résumé of the significant work which his academy has also done in connexion with the history of the origin of agriculture in the world.

In industry, as well as in agriculture, the Soviet Union lays great emphasis on adequate facilities for research. It is reported that in 1930 there were established 72 industrial scientific research institutes with 83 branches, while factory laboratories now run into thousands. The technologists of our party spent some time in visiting these institutes, but I did not myself have time to do so, and therefore, in spite of their obvious importance, will do no more than mention their existence.

To anyone who believes that the salvation of human society depends ultimately on the intelligent application of scientific methods to social problems, and that the gross economic muddle which today is precipitating unprecedented crises all over the world can only be straightened out by a strict scientific control of production and distribution on a large scale basis, the attitude of modern Socialist Russia to scientific research and application is of fundamental significance and must be taken into account when estimating what is likely to be the future influence of the Soviet Union on the progress of civilization in general. It is not a little striking that in Russia, where in pre-revolutionary times there was perhaps less organized scientific research than in any other large European country, the organization of research and the application of scientific methods under centralized control should today be apparently progressing on a larger scale than anywhere else in the world. Russia is essentially a country of contrasts. This must inevitably be the case when it is realized that an astonishingly abrupt transition is being made from what was little more than a mediaeval civilization to a social system which in the eyes of many people outside Russia appears distinctly futuristic. Nowhere are these contrasts more obtrusive, perhaps, than in Moscow, where one is constantly meeting with scenes and incidents that serve to emphasize the intermingling of primitive and ultra-modern culture. I have tried to put into writing a few of the impressions which I received on my short visit to Soviet Russia. As I emphasized at the beginning of this article, these impressions are based on what obviously must have been very superficial observations made during a brief and hurried tour. In spite of these disadvantages, I am glad to have had the opportunity of seeing modern Russia first-hand, for I have had a personal glimpse, however fleeting, of an experiment in social reorganization which is being carried out on an unprecedented scale. What the outcome of the experiment may ultimately be, I cannot attempt to judge, but I imagine that it deserves the attention of all those who may be interested in problems of sociology, even if only from the academic standpoint.

CHAPTER 6

OXFORD RETROSPECTIONS

WHEN I submitted my candidature for the vacant Chair of Anatomy at Oxford University, I did so with some feelings of misgiving. I enjoyed working amongst old colleagues at St. Thomas's Hospital, and I had become much attached to our house and garden at Digswell. But the removal to Oxford was no doubt a step up in the academic ladder, and there were many pleasing amenities to look forward to, including a Fellowship of Hertford College. I was duly elected to the Chair and we moved to Oxford in 1934. After a preliminary two years during which we rented a house, we were fortunate enough to buy what I have always thought to be the most attractive of the houses in Belbroughton Road. The road itself was also attractive with its enticing gardens; its charm has been commemorated by John Betjeman in his poem 'Spring Morning in North Oxford'—

> Belbroughton Road is bonny, and pinkly bursts the spray
> Of prunus and forsythia across the public way,
> For a full spring-tide of blossom seethed and departed hence,
> Leaving land-locked pools of jonquils by sunny garden fence.

The Anatomy Department at Oxford was a good deal more spacious than I had up to then been accustomed to, but at first sight not quite spacious enough in its available accommodation for the sort of teaching and research facilities I hoped to develop. But it had possibilities and, in order to realize these, I had some initial difficulties to overcome that involved me in animated (though, I am happy to say, not really acrimonious) tussles with some of my colleagues of other departments who did not altogether agree with my plans. My predecessor was

Professor Arthur Thomson who had been in charge of the Department for almost fifty years—he had retired in 1933. He was an able exponent of human embryology and physical anthropology in both of which subjects he had made useful contributions, but he abandoned his embryological studies after describing in detail what he believed to be the earliest human embryo known at that time—a simple cluster of cells as yet undifferentiated into contrasting elements. When, after two years of intensive study, his substantial monograph on this specimen was sent to a scientific journal for publication, the editorial advisers suggested, rightly as it turned out, that the supposed early embryo was really nothing more than a blocked uterine gland filled with cellular débris. This curious error of Arthur Thomson's led to some unhappy correspondence between him and the editorial advisers, the details of which came to my attention when, on taking up my appointment at Oxford, I had to sift through all the papers and files that he had left behind in the Department of Anatomy. The correspondence made melancholy reading because I realized what a shock it must have been to Arthur Thomson when his astonishing mistake was pointed out to him. He was a man of genial and kindly temperament, and he had achieved much in building up his Department from the brick and iron-roofed sheds that housed it when he was appointed in 1885 to the well-planned stone building that he designed and completed in 1893. Following the unfortunate incident of the 'early embryo', he no longer took any interest in embryology and focussed his attention on physical anthropology, particularly on craniometric studies of skulls. Thus it came about that the only room in the Anatomy Department that could possibly be converted into a teaching laboratory I found to be occupied by about three thousand human skulls displayed in glass-fronted cases. These made quite an imposing array, but in fact they had come to be very rarely used for study and, although they represented many different races from different parts of the world, there were too few from any one geographical region to be of effective use for measurements designed for the statistical analysis of contrasting racial characters. On the other hand, in the Natural History Museum in South Kensington there was housed a much larger collection of some ten thousand human skulls, and I argued that if the Oxford collections were to be added to the latter they would be much more usefully available to any student who might wish to make a study of racial differences in craniological features. Further, if this were done, the room occupied by them in my department could be converted into a much needed laboratory. There arose what I used to call 'The Battle of the Skulls', for this proposal was rather strongly opposed by some of my anthropological colleagues in the University. But the force of my argument did finally prevail, and the skulls were transferred on 'permanent loan' to the Natural History Museum. The flurry of controversy over these skulls gave rise to a good deal of amusement among other members of the University, for the reason that years previously they had been accommodated in the Museum of Zoology and Comparative Anatomy under the care of Ray Lankester, and my predecessor, Arthur Thomson, had been engaged in quite a lengthy struggle with him to get the collection transferred to the Department of Anatomy where he thought they should more appropriately be placed. Mine was thus really the second 'Battle of the Skulls', but in reverse.

When I arrived in Oxford I found one most curious feature in the Department of Anatomy that truly astonished me. The women medical students were segregated from the men for their practical dissection of the human body. According to the authors of *A Short History of Anatomical Teaching in Oxford* Professor Thomson had decided, when women medical students first appeared in the University, that they 'must dissect

in a room apart from the men, and should only receive instruction in surface anatomy down to the level of the umbilicus'.
Whether this is a strictly true account I do not know, but at
any rate a separate dissecting-room for women was built on
the top floor of the north side of the Anatomy Department,
the cost of construction being met by a private benefaction,
and there was also provided accommodation for a woman
anatomist to supervise their work. I decided that it was proper,
as well as convenient, to transfer the girls down to the main
dissecting-room; there they worked happily enough with the
boys, neither distracting the other from serious attention to
their studies. This set free the women's dissecting-room and
ancillary accommodation for conversion into the additional
research laboratories that I needed for my staff.

I found still further room to accommodate expansion of
work in the Department in a spacious 'studio' that my predecessor had built on the top of the south side of the building.
He was an accomplished water-colour painter; and he also
published an excellent book on *Anatomy for Art Students* with
photographic illustrations. Accordingly, he built the studio for
his photographic work as well as for his less academic painting.
It was exceptionally well lighted and well ventilated, and attached to it was a small dark-room for developing and printing
photographs. It proved in many ways to be most convenient for
conversion into an 'animal house' to accommodate experimental
animals, while the dark-room was readily transformed into a
kitchen where the food for the animals could be prepared.
This change-over was planned and accomplished without
difficulty.

Another small problem remained to be solved; the entrance
hall in the Department at that time was adorned with life-size
plaster casts of Venus de Milo, Antinous, the Fighting Gladiator,
and Goodsir's representation of a dead and partially dissected
human body. These, I suppose, had been thought to be an

appropriate introduction to a Department of the University in which human anatomy was studied. But I did not feel they were in harmony with current trends in anatomical teaching and research, and they occupied a good deal of space needed for other purposes. Two of the statues, also, were already disfigured by missing fingers and broken noses. I was in something of a quandary in deciding how to get rid of these plaster casts, for they had originally been donated to the Department of Anatomy in 1893 by Sir Henry Acland who was then Regius Professor of Medicine at Oxford. In my dilemma I consulted the University Registrar, Mr (later Sir Douglas) Veale; I had sought his advice on several occasions during my first year or two at Oxford on the best procedure to follow without the need to ask for formal permission through a succession of boards and committees, and he was always anxious, and usually able, to help me towards the realization of my plans for the development of my Department by methods of short-circuiting such bodies. I owe him much for his helpful advice, and on this occasion it was, as usual, good. He suggested that I should remove the plaster statuary down to hidden recesses in the basement, and, if after six months nobody made any mention of their disappearance, I should then just have them broken up. This I did, no particular notice was taken by anybody, and that was the end of them.

The teaching and technical staff of the Anatomy Department on my arrival in 1934 was very small. There was a Reader in Anatomy, Dr Blake Odgers, senior to me in years and always helpful and co-operative even though, as I suspect, he may not have entirely approved of my innovations in matters of organization. Dr Alice Carleton was a University Demonstrator and had gained an exceptionally high reputation for her teaching ability. For some years she had also been practising as a dermatologist, so that she was not able to give all the attention to the Department which might be expected of a University post, though she showed considerable ability in the programmes of anatomical research which she did carry out. I soon discovered, rather to my surprise at the time, that divided attention between Departmental and other duties in Oxford was quite common, for some University Demonstrators or Lecturers who were also Fellows of a College often devoted a good deal of their time to tutorial work in their College and to College administration. My surprise at these dual roles was short-lived, however, for I had not realized all the advantages to student life that the College system has to offer; I had not experienced anything of the kind during my years in London, and it certainly seemed to work very well to the advantage of the undergraduates.

The Reader in Physical Anthropology in my Department was Dr Dudley Buxton, a man of wide knowledge in several branches of anthropological science. So far as concerns physical anthropology, however, he tended to cling to traditional methods such as craniometry which by that time were beginning to be superseded by a more dynamic approach to the subject. But he did not demur when I had to take up some of the accommodation in the Department that previously he had rightly regarded as his own territory, in order to provide the space I needed for experimental studies which I and some members of my staff wanted to undertake, and which I hoped would attract visiting research workers to Oxford. Within a few months of taking up my appointment I was able to add to my teaching staff two junior demonstrators. One of these was Dr (later Sir Solly) Zuckerman who was of considerable help to me in the reorganizing and replanning of my Department. His main scientific interest at that time was in the field of endocrinology with particular reference to the sex hormones, and he soon became engaged in a study of the factors that regulate the menstrual rhythm in baboons. I well remember that there was natural consternation among some of my colleagues when these ferocious looking creatures were imported into a rather unsuitable room in the basement of the Department where they were for a time accommodated in large cages. Zuckerman remained a member of my staff for ten years; active in research himself, he had an unusual capacity for organizing teams of young research workers concentrating their attention on problems of common interest. In view of the success of his scientific career in later years, I feel happy that I was able to grant him the facilities he needed for his earlier endocrinological work in my Department, for it was this work that gave him a foothold in the long ladder of success that followed.

In 1934 the technical staff of the Anatomy Department was as limited as the teaching and research staff. Its senior member was Mr Chesterman on whom devolved many and diverse duties—vicarious secretarial responsibilities (I had no full-time secretary either for my personal or for departmental work), supervising all the formalities related to the accession and disposal of cadavers used for the practical dissection courses, keeping the accounts that had to be prepared annually for the University Chest, ordering routine supplies for the Department, doing laboratory work such as the cutting and staining of microscopical sections, assisting at lectures and classes, and from time to time undertaking microphotography with the use of an antiquated apparatus that required a good deal of time-consuming adjustments before a satisfactory microphotograph could be obtained, and so forth. I never quite understood how he managed to accomplish all these duties, for he always seemed to move about with a leisurely imperturbability. I was much indebted to Mr Chesterman for helping to initiate me into the mysteries of administrating an Oxford University Department, and also for his technical assistance in my research work. But I also had my personal technical assistant whom I had trained in laboratory work at St. Thomas's Hospital when he was still a young boy fresh from school, and whom I brought to Oxford with me.

There was in the Department a small workshop equipped with tools and apparatus required for carpentry and a modest degree of metal work; this was in the charge of a highly skilled craftsman, Mr Peade, a man of exceptional intelligence as well as of unusual technical competence. Much of the successful research work that later emanated from the Anatomy Department could not have been achieved but for his advice and ingenuity in designing and constructing special types of laboratory apparatus.

One other man whom I found on the technical staff was an old ex-naval rating who, with the help of Mr Chesterman, was responsible for embalming the cadavers for dissection. But he had other duties also; he acted as a general 'cleaner' in the Department, and he had also to make and keep up the coal fires that were required to warm most of the staff rooms. The fact that open coal fires were still in use in research laboratories seemed to me to be a peculiar anomaly, and more than anything else, I think, it made me realize that at least some parts of the University had not yet emerged from the end of the previous century. But this old custom had its advantages by again providing extra accommodation, for a spacious room in the basement was used as a coal cellar, and, having replaced the open grates by gas fires, I was able to convert this room into yet another useful research laboratory.

I have mentioned that my appointment to the Chair of Anatomy at Oxford was associated with a Fellowship of Hertford College. This custom at the University of allocating the various professorial chairs to fellowships among the various Colleges was a happy custom, for it brought newly elected professors without delay into the community of College life with all the intimate associations arising from it. Herein Oxford professors had at that time a great advantage over those at Cambridge, for there new professors might have to wait for several years before they were nominated for election to a College Fellowship, and, until that happened, they naturally felt they were not fully integrated into the University organization as a whole. I felt it a great privilege to be a Fellow of Hertford College and to take an active part in the business of its Governing Body. Although the present foundation of the College, properly speaking, only dates from 1874, some of its buildings had a long history within the University under the name of Hart Hall, mention of which first occurs in a conveyance made by Elias de Hertford in 1301, and later under the name of Magdalen Hall. Among its worthies of the past were the philosopher Thomas Hobbes, William Tyndale whose translation provided the foundation for the authorized version of the bible, and Thomas Sydenham, perhaps the most distinguished physician of the seventeenth century.

In the late summer and early autumn of 1934 I occasionally found myself wandering in a meditative mood through the Colleges and their gardens, and at such times I seemed, as it were, to imbibe into the inner recesses of my mind something of the spirit and traditions that had grown up with the centuries of Oxford scholarship. Compared with London there was an atmosphere quite remarkably reposeful and inspiring in the quietness of the quadrangles and gardens enclosed by ancient buildings. In such surroundings, little changed, there wandered three hundred years ago illustrious men whose names have come down to posterity and still continue to be associated with their achievements. I thought of William Harvey, the discoverer of the circulation of the blood, who was for a short time with Charles I in Oxford during the Civil War, and briefly Warden of Merton College in 1646 at the time he was studying the development of the embryo chick. I thought also, of the eminent anatomists Richard Lower (who has been credited with the distinction of being the first to carry out a blood transfusion) and Thomas Willis, of Robert Boyle the chemist who is still commemorated by 'Boyle's Law' (i.e. that the volume of a gas varies inversely as the pressure) and who aided his contemporary anatomists by investigating chemical methods for preserving anatomical material from putrefaction, and of Christopher Wren who, quite apart from his architectural feats in Oxford represented particularly by the Sheldonian Theatre and Tom Tower, engaged in physiological experiments and drew the illustrations for Thomas Willis's classical work *Cerebri Anatome* published in 1664. I could persuade myself that in my imagination I saw such intellectual giants strolling along Broad Street and around the College gardens, and that I listened to them discussing and discoursing on the scientific and philosophical problems which interested them in those days. A feeling of reverence for great traditions of the past has always seemed to me to provide a most powerful incentive for seeking to uphold them into the present—it suffuses the mind with a glow of warm excitement urging on efforts to make the present worthy of the past. Such indeed was my own experience when I first introduced myself to the University of Oxford and sensed its intellectual climate rich with history of the years gone by.

On my election to a Fellowship of Hertford College I found that the Senior Common Room was then a small and distinguished, but academically rather limited, community. Apart from the Principal there were fourteen Fellows, but for a long time it was a static community, for I remained the junior Fellow for no less than fifteen years. There were no other scientists represented on the Governing Body of the College except Dr Ferrar of mathematical repute, but there were some notable representatives of what are termed, in the broadest sense, the Humanities. I think particularly of J. D. Denniston, an eminent classical scholar whose sudden and untimely death occurred in 1949; Dr T. S. Boase, an authority on the history of art who later became President of Magdalen College; Felix Markham, whose intimate studies of Napoleonic times are well known; James Meade, a young economist who was destined to become the distinguished Professor of Political Economy at Cambridge; and John Armstrong, a mediaeval historian of note. The Principal was Dr Cruttwell, recognized for his brilliance as a modern historian. He was addicted to the mild eccentricities that are commonly associated with Oxford intellectuals; in manner he tended to be somewhat abrupt, and at first I found it difficult to open up a sustained conversation with him on general topics. But later on I came to know him well, and his tragic death in 1941 shortly after I went to see him in a nursing home was a particularly distressing episode.

There are some who seem to think that the Senior Common Room conversation after dinner is consistently sparkling, creative, and fertile in discussion of problems of wide interest. Sparkling it often is, but it seemed to me that serious and sustained disputation aimed at sorting out conflicting opinions in order, if possible, to arrive at an agreed solution occasionally tended to be frustrated by the more frivolous-minded members of a College who gave the impression that they were interested rather in winning a laugh by seeking for the *mot juste* than in resolutely pursuing a discussion in logical sequence. This type of 'argument by guffaw' (as I used to term it in my own thoughts) I found somewhat irritating, and certainly not very illuminating, but it was more than counterbalanced by the conversational brilliance on other occasions. Naturally, it is not to be expected that Senior Common Room conversation is consistently brilliant; it fluctuates quite considerably in its interests and there are evenings when it is frankly dull and uninteresting. In the convivial atmosphere of guest nights at Hertford College, or of commemorative dinners at other Colleges that were commonly attended by a number of academic virtuosos, it was particularly then that sparks began to fly from crackling conversations filled with witticisms and spontaneous epigrams. Such nights, sometimes carried on to the early hours of the morning, provided an intellectual revelry hardly to be surpassed by any other form of entertainment. Looking back, I think the two most brilliant conversationalists of my time were the Warden of Wadham, Sir Maurice Bowra, and the Principal of Brasenose, the late Dr Stallybrass. It was indeed a joy to listen to their epigrammatic commentaries on an astonishing diversity of topics.

Although I was able to increase the staff of the Anatomy Department to a limited extent between 1934 and 1939, the annual grant from the University for the running of the Department remained pitifully small; I had in large part to rely on annual grants from outside sources to maintain a reasonable level of research activity, and the recurrent need to make applications for these grants (and to justify them by our research achievements) took up a good deal of my time as well as involving some degree of perennial anxiety. When, therefore, I was offered the Chair of Anatomy at University College, London, early in 1939 I was tempted to accept this. But my wife and I decided to do so only after the most painful heart-searchings. Oxford had many very pleasant amenities and we made a number of good friends there. On the other hand, at that time University College had what was regarded as the premier Department of Anatomy in England, well endowed and with excellent laboratory accommodation and an ample staff. Further, the prospects for its greater development were very favourable. Having made our decision to return to London, we began to look around for a house in the country suitable for ready access to University College by train. Then the Second World War broke out, only a few weeks before I was due to take up my new appointment, and the Provost of University College suggested that our arrangements should be cancelled and the appointment reconsidered anew at the end of the war. This proved to be a fortunate circumstance for me, fortunate from several points of view. For one thing, if the war had started a few weeks later I should have found myself evacuated with my new Department to temporary accommodation outside London with only limited and makeshift facilities for teaching and research. For another thing during the war the Department of Anatomy at Oxford received very substantial grants for research into war-time problems, and these made it possible for me to increase and extend my laboratory and workshop equipment to such an extent that the research facilities at the end of the war were far better than they had been before. I found, too, that by then I had become integrated into the life of the University with much greater intimacy, and this was accompanied by a deeper sense of friendship with my academic colleagues and a still greater appreciation of all that the University of Oxford stands for. I suppose most will agree that, in moving from one community or institution associated with certain traditions to another with quite a different organization and a different set of traditions, it does take some time before you are able to identify yourself heart and soul with your new environment. Certainly I found this to be the case in my first year or two at Oxford.

Apart from other considerations, no doubt one of the main advantages that I gained in Oxford (as compared with those available to me in my previous positions in London) derived from the fact that my department was immediately surrounded by other scientific Departments whose directors were men of exceptionally high distinction, and whose acquaintance I valued not only for academic reasons but also for their personal friendship. In charge of the Physiology Department was Sir Charles Sherrington—in his time one of the most eminent (more probably true to say, *the* most eminent) of neurophysiologists. He was quick to offer me laboratory facilities in his

Department for my neurological studies until such time as I could build and equip my own research laboratories. Sir Rudolph Peters was the Professor of Biochemistry, and, a year after my arrival, Howard (later Lord) Florey, of penicillin fame, was appointed to the Professorship of Pathology. Sir Robert Robinson headed the Dyson Perrins Department of Organic Chemistry, Sir Cyril Hinshelwood was Professor of Physical Chemistry, and in charge of the Zoology Department was Professor Goodrich (not only a distinguished zoologist but also a surprisingly good water-colour artist). Professor Sollas, then of an advanced age, was the Professor of Geology who, apart from his purely geological work, had developed an interest in problems related to fossil man. In charge of the Pitt Rivers Museum, directly adjacent to my own Department, was Dr Balfour, an eminent exponent of ethnology and comparative technology. It is worthy of note that Robinson, Hinshelwood and Florey all became in their turn Presidents of the Royal Society, and all became Nobel laureates.

Besides my professorial colleagues, there were of course many members of the staff of their Departments who were also distinguished scientists in their own particular fields of study, a number of whom in later years achieved pre-eminence for their scientific work. Day-to-day contacts and conversations with them enlarged my horizon of scientific knowledge very considerably and were particularly useful in those marginal fields of research closely akin to my own studies. Guest nights at Hertford College, and being entertained from time to time in other Colleges, brought me the acquaintance of authorities on many subjects apart from those of strictly scientific interest —men of literary fame, historians, philosophers, economists, sociologists, legal experts, administrators of international repute, and so forth. To all these I owe much for the stimulating and informative ideas that they conveyed to me in casual conversations.

One curious incident that occurred three or four years after my arrival in Oxford I recall most vividly because of its bizarre nature—the appearance of a 'poltergeist' in my Department. I call it a 'poltergeist' because it manifested all the sorts of phenomenon commonly attributed to such visitations. During a period of a few weeks we would find on arriving in the morning at the Department that cupboards had been smashed open, keys had disappeared, laboratory benches had been deliberately cut with a sharp knife, and laboratory apparatus had been hurled about on the floor. All this made no sense, for nothing of value had been stolen. Naturally enough, it led to a disturbed and rather tense atmosphere in the Department, for we all tended to develop suspicions of deranged activities affecting some other member of the Department. During this uncomfortable episode, I used to go down to the Department in the dead of night and wait, hoping to catch the culprit, but unsuccessfully. Finally, one cupboard was found broken open, and in it a pencilled message intimating threats to one of the members of the technical staff. Following this, I constructed a paragraph including here and there all the words of which the message was composed and I summoned every member of the staff to my room to write out the paragraph to my dictation. By such means I discovered the culprit—the last person I should have suspected. He was a nice young lad, well-liked by his co-workers and particularly assiduous in carrying out his duties in the Department. He admitted his responsibility for all the odd happenings that had occurred, and returned all the keys that he had removed. Naturally, I had to ask him to leave, for his own sake as well as for the peace of mind of other members of the staff. But his behaviour turned out to be no more than a temporary aberration of adolescence, for he subsequently had a good record of service in the army during the Second World War, became happily married, and for long occupied a secure position as an industrial worker. From time to time there appear in the more sensational press accounts of 'poltergeists' for which it is assumed there is no explanation except those of a purely psychical nature. After my own experience I have become more non-commital about these so-called paranormal phenomena, and, indeed, I know that many, or perhaps all, of those so reported have proved to be the result of ingenious tricks. No doubt the most famous of these cases is that of Borley Rectory in Essex, which puzzled many reputable authorities for quite a number of years. The final exposure of this 'poltergeist' was recorded in a book, *The Haunting of Borley Rectory*, by E. J. Dingwall and others published in 1956. It appears that a certain Harry Price, self-styled Director of the National Laboratory of Psychical Research, went down to Borley to investigate the phenomena, and, as he had previously exposed the fraudulent nature of similar cases, his integrity was naturally not questioned. But when he arrived to carry out his investigations, the poltergeist phenomena became even more intensified than they had been previously. Price wrote a book describing his observations and referred therein to 'the most extraordinary and best documented case' in the annals of psychical research. It is also remarkable that two eminent jurists (and here I reproduce quotations from Dingwall's book) were evidently quite convinced by the evidence. The late Sir Albion Richardson, K.C., in remarking on Price's book about Borley Rectory, wrote, 'The evidence which he has collected of the phenomena which appeared there is as conclusive as human testimony can be and is admirably marshalled. I have not met anyone who has read the book—and it is mainly with legal friends of long experience in the weighing and sifting of evidence that I have discussed it (many of them, like myself, previously sceptical)—who has not been satisfied that the manifestations therein disclosed are proved by the evidence, to the point of moral certainty.' The other jurist, the late Sir Ernest Jelf, similarly expressed his opinion that the case for the paranormal character of the phenomena reported by Price was very strong, stronger indeed 'than most of us could ever have believed possible before we had read the book', and that, on the face of it, it was difficult 'to understand what cross-examination could possibly shake it'. And yet, as it turned out later, there seems little doubt that it was Harry Price himself who actually fabricated at least some of the evidence assumed to be the result of psychical manifestations! I mention this remarkable case to demonstrate that even the wisest, most intelligent, and most experienced of men (and not only jurists but sometimes scientists also) may be led to accept as valid the evidence for extrasensory phenomena that, at the time, may otherwise seem to them to be inexplicable in other terms.

If the growth of my Department at Oxford and of its teaching and research staff was but slowly progressive during my first few years there, it developed a sudden spurt of activity when the war began in 1939. For one thing, the whole of the Anatomy School of St. Thomas's Hospital was evacuated to Oxford, and accommodation and facilities had to be provided for their teaching; this of course added considerably to my administrative responsibilities. But, apart from this, research activities were rapidly stepped up to explore the many problems that were posed by civilian defence and by the fighting forces in the field. The research staff in the Department was thus greatly augmented by the recruitment of personnel seconded from the forces and elsewhere (including two members of the Free French Forces); for their accommodation additional rooms had to be provided, and a hutted laboratory was also erected immediately adjacent to the main Department for this purpose. Some of the research was focussed on the treatment of war injuries. For example, we investigated the potentialities for repair following damage to the central nervous system, that is, the brain and spinal cord. It is well known that peripheral nerves, that is to say, the nerves that supply muscles, skin,

CPE L

blood-vessels and so forth, can undergo quite rapid regeneration after they have been severed by a deep cut, but for some reason or another bundles of nerve fibres within the central nervous system seem to lack this capacity for repair. However, it had been reported some years previously that under certain experimental conditions regeneration of nerve fibres in the brain following their interruption by wounding lesions *could* be induced. It seemed important, therefore, to investigate this matter more closely. But, unfortunately, our own studies, with more carefully controlled experiments, did not confirm the results of earlier investigators. Newly growing nerve fibres were indeed found at the site of the lesions, but they proved to be the result of the ingrowth of peripheral nerve fibres from the membranes covering the surface of the brain, or from peripheral nerve fibres concerned with the innervation of local blood vessels. Moreover, a peripheral nerve, such as the facial nerve, inserted into the substance of the brain through an incision, was found to regenerate and proliferate there with great vigour, while the *intrinsic* nerve fibres of the brain immediately surrounding the implanted nerve and interrupted by the incision remained quite inactive. This was a disappointing result, for it seemed to show that the intrinsic nerve fibres of the brain (at any rate in mammals) are incapable of repair to the extent that this can lead to a reconstitution of normal function—a conclusion that was in accordance with innumerable clinical observations on patients in whom tracts of nerve fibres in the brain and spinal cord had been severed by injury or disease. It is interesting to note, however, that since the war it has been claimed by some American observers that some degree of regeneration of nerve fibres in the mammalian central nervous system can occur if a local inflammatory reaction is induced at the site of an injury, but it remains exceedingly doubtful whether this can proceed so far as to lead to any useful functional restoration. In other words, if a bundle of nerve fibres in the brain or spinal cord is interrupted by an injury, restoration of function is not to be expected. And this unfortunately applies also to the optic nerve of the eye, for this is not a 'nerve' in the usual sense of the term—it is really a nerve tract of the brain that becomes extruded from the latter in the course of embryonic development.

Other work was carried out, under the direction of my colleague, Dr Graham Weddell, on the mode of repair of sensory nerves to the skin that had been cut by wounding injuries, with particular reference to the part played by the fine cells that ensheathe each of the nerve fibres, and to the recovery of sensation in those areas of the skin that had become numbed by the interruption of the nerves that normally supply them. When a peripheral nerve is cut, all the nerve fibres beyond the level of the injury undergo complete degeneration, but those above the level send out new sprouts that grow down (at the rate of about two millimetres a day) until they re-innervate the area of the skin involved. But recovery of sensation is a gradual process because, as it was established by these experiments, each single sensory spot is supplied by a number of different nerve fibres that approach it from different directions and some may take longer than others to arrive at their destination. Consequently, there is a temporary phase of *partial* innervation of the sensory spots during which the sensation of the affected skin area remains crude and uncertain. Not until each spot receives its full, multiple, innervation from regenerated nerve fibres can full sensory restoration be expected. Another interesting point that emerged from these studies is that a desensitized area of skin may become invaded by sprouts from normal cutaneous nerve fibres in immediately adjacent areas that invade its margins. Thus, the shrinkage of a numbed area of skin following the interruption of a main nerve that supplies it does not necessarily mean that any of the fibres of this particular nerve have yet reached their final destination.

Yet other studies of nerve injuries involving motor nerves to muscles leading to their paralysis were concerned with the use of what is called electromyography as a diagnostic agent for tracing the course of regeneration of the motor nerve fibres into the muscles and the restoration of their function. When fine electrodes are inserted into a normal muscle, the electrical activity that can be recorded is quite characteristic, but when the muscle is denervated, that is to say when the nerve is cut and it becomes paralysed, the electrical activity of the muscular tissue changes its pattern. Again, when the regenerating motor fibres of the muscle begin to make functional contact with some of the muscle fibres, the electrical activity betrays their presence. It will be realized, therefore, that this method, applied clinically to patients, may be of the greatest service in prognosticating the chances of a favourable recovery.

Another of our war-time research problems concerned an enquiry into the reparative capacity of muscle tissue itself following direct injury by deep wounds. Here we made the interesting observation that, provided the wound is not severely lacerating and followed by the formation of dense scar tissue, dead muscle fibres can be replaced by the growth of new fibres much more readily than had been supposed. If, for instance, a blood-vessel supplying part of a muscle is interrupted, the devascularized fibres undergo a necrotic dissolution. But new fibres sprout from the ends of uninjured fibres and grow along to replace the dead elements. It appeared, indeed, that muscle tissue is not able to survive for more than a short time if it is deprived of its blood supply. This demonstration led on to a careful study of the pattern of blood-vessels that supply individual muscles in the human body, a matter of some importance to the operating surgeon, for it became obvious that he should have a clear picture of the pattern of blood-vessels supplying a muscle so that he can carefully avoid cutting any of them.

No doubt the more immediately important research work carried out in the Department of Anatomy was that related to problems of attack and defence. Much of this, of course, was secret work the results of which were issued in confidential documents. For example, the Royal Naval Personnel Research Committee of the Medical Research Council required anatomical and physiological data that would help in the design of seating and sighting apparatus, and in determining the optimal position of hand levers and foot pedals that would allow them to be operated with maximum efficiency and minimum fatigue over long periods of time. These investigations involved anthropometric surveys, and the study of the natural movements of various joints so that the controls of a machine could be as accurately as possible geared to them. In other words— they were problems of 'fitting the machine to the man'. The investigations into these problems were in principle straightforward enough, but they involved a considerable amount of work, including the systematic study of a large number of individuals of different body proportions. But the results were rewarding for they led to a redesigning of equipment that certainly enhanced the efficiency and the operational accuracy of the service personnel making use of it. Incidentally, investigations of this kind, aimed at maximizing efficiency and minimizing fatigue by accurately gearing the controls of a machine to the natural movements of the operator working it —a matter of humanizing the machine rather than mechanizing the man, as I have expressed it—came later to assume considerable importance in relation to industrial problems of peacetime.

The study of the effects of blast on the living body and the study of the damage incurred by soft tissues and bone produced by missiles of different sizes travelling at different velocities were carried out under the supervision of my colleague Solly Zuckerman, and this naturally led on to the investigation of protective measures such as body armour and air raid shelters, the statistical analysis of air-raid casualties, the assessment of bomb damage to buildings, and the analysis of casualties incurred in actual fighting. All this extensive work, which came under the heading of 'operational research', was highly important for the prosecution of the war, and Zuckerman was to become an outstanding authority on similar problems.

These years of war-time research stand out as a sort of promontory of particularly engrossing activity during my Oxford days. But, more than that, they led on at the end of the war to a marked expansion of peace-time activities. Our laboratory and workshop equipment had been considerably augmented and improved, and the research staff of the Department had also increased in numbers. And there were changes in the staff of which the most notable were the appointment of Solly Zuckerman to the Chair of Anatomy at Birmingham University (one of a number of my staff who came to be promoted to professorships in various universities), and the appointment of Dr J. S. Weiner as Reader in Physical Anthropology in my Department, replacing Dr Dudley Buxton who had died some years previously. The accession of Dr Weiner (later to become a professor in the University of London) was particularly welcome, for he played a most important part in reorientating the curriculum in physical anthropology and liberating it from some of its traditional and outmoded concepts. As the result of his work the subject became much more dynamic in its approach to modern problems whereas for some time it had become rather static in its educational content. During the war he had been engaged in London on a study of the factors determining the climatic adaptation of the human body to extremes of temperature, humidity and so forth, with special reference to the needs of the fighting forces who had to contend with climatic extremes. When he came to Oxford he continued these studies, and later applied them to problems of peace-time activities in various industrial projects at home and abroad. This field of research, combined with our continued enquiries on problems of 'fitting the machine to the man', led to the establishment of a Medical Research Council Unit in the Department, whose main objective was the study of man in his working environment. I was appointed the Honorary Director of this Unit, but my main duties were of an administrative kind—a necessary appointment since the Unit had to be integrated into the general organization of my Department. My office of Director was far from being a sine-cure, however, for I had the ultimate responsibility for its continuing success, and on occasion it raised difficult problems of personnel that I had to try to resolve. Nevertheless, it did pursue a reasonably successful career until my retirement in 1962, when the Unit was transferred to London under the competent Directorship of Professor Weiner and with the title of the Environmental Physiology Research Unit.

Towards the end of the war there occurred a singular episode that still stands our rather starkly in my memory. It was an episode that at the time made me feel very uncomfortable, but which later assumed a somewhat humorous aspect. I was then, with some other senior members of the University, an active member of the Society for Cultural Relations with Soviet Russia, our ally during the war. A Russian doctor, Professor Sarkisov, was in England acting in liaison with our own medical officials of the Red Cross, and he had brought with him a film designed to illustrate the efficiency of the organization of the Russian medical services in the fighting zone. It was suggested that he should show this film to a public audience in Oxford. Now, I had heard that it might not be altogether suitable for a lay audience because some of the sequences were too blatantly 'medical' in their presentation of the subject. I was not able myself to have a pre-view of the film for I was up in London when Sarkisov arrived in Oxford, so I asked the secretary of the S.C.R., a layman himself, to have it run through before it was publicly exhibited. He reported to me that it contained nothing that might affect the susceptibilities of a non-medical audience. Accordingly, I arranged for the film to be shown in a large lecture theatre in one of the University Departments. The theatre was packed with an eager audience. The film started off with shots of wounded soldiers being picked up and transported back from the front line in motor ambulances and aeroplanes. So far so good. But then it began to show 'close-ups' of the surgical treatment of wounds in base hospitals. This proved too much for some members of the audience. First one fainted, then another, and then several more. As the chairman of the meeting I began to feel very uncertain how I should best proceed to meet this awkward situation. The first reel of the film was approaching its end when someone ran down the gangway to where I was sitting and whispered to me in great urgency that the cinema operator himself had fainted. I rushed to the back of the theatre, tore up the winding staircase leading to the projection room, and found the projectionist stretched out senseless on the floor. As I have said, the first reel was nearing its end, and of course we did not know how to switch it off. However, we managed to revive the man in time and supported him while he turned off the right switch. The lights came on and I had a hurried consultation with the S.C.R. secretary on the advisability of continuing with the show, but he assured me that the next reel was quite innocuous. I conveyed this message to the audience while apologizing for the disturbing effects of the first reel. The lights went out and we started on the second reel. Then, to my dismay, this began to show 'close-ups' of brain operations! However, by now the general atmosphere had changed, and the audience began to laugh uproariously, presumably because the film belied so ridiculously the assurances I had given them. But my anxieties were not over. The entrance hall of the theatre looked like a casualty clearing station, with a number of 'patients' still lying prostrate and looking very unwell and I had to attend to them, with the help of some of my associates already with them, until they were sufficiently revived to make their way home. Professor Sarkisov seemed to be rather amused at this reaction of multiple fainting. But no doubt it was really a case of one highly susceptible person fainting and then, by a sort of psychological 'contagion' others following suit. I recollect this kind of thing happening when I was at school; if one of the boys fell into a faint in chapel for some quite adequate reason, frequently two or three others would faint also for no reason at all except as an expression of the well recognized phenomenon of sympathetic reaction.

During the years following the end of the war, the work of teaching and research progressed evenly and smoothly. I had been fortunate in gathering a highly competent staff, augmented in almost continuous succession by post-graduate students from abroad who stayed for two or three years to acquaint themselves with our teaching and research methods. Most of these took an advanced degree, usually a doctorate, at Oxford, and a few eventually came to take up a permanent appointment in the Department. It is not practicable to list all these, but I would particularly like to mention two of them, Tom Powell and Max Cowan, both of whom became distinguished as experimental neurologists and to whom I owed much for their stimulating collaboration and advice. Dr Weddell became the Reader in Human Anatomy and pursued his studies of peripheral nerves with special reference to problems of cutaneous sensation, and he continued to attract research students who from time to time sought to learn his methods of demonstrating fine nerve fibres by special staining techniques. Apart from the work of the Medical Research Council Unit, which was now directed towards peace-time problems, and much of which was accomplished by the constant use of a climatic chamber in which the temperature, humidity and air current could be controlled so as to simulate climatic environments normally found in many parts of the world, the research activities in the Department were spread over wide fields of enquiry—neurological studies with particular reference to the structure and functions of the brain, microscopical techniques, patterns of blood supply to various tissues and organs, cellular anatomy, the structure and growth of muscle and tendon, anthropological studies of modern man, studies of fossil man and fossil apes, and so forth.

On the teaching side we were eager to introduce some reform in the curriculum by eliminating much of the factual details and minutiae of gross topographical anatomy that medical students had for many years been required to memorize for examination purposes. Considering that not more than three per cent of our students would ever be required to undertake operations of major surgery, why, we asked ourselves, should they be compelled to learn and memorize all the trivial and unimportant branches of blood-vessels, the precise relationships of a deeply situated muscle and all its minor attachments, the exact course and position of many small nerves, or the details of the shape and joint surfaces of small bones such as those of the wrist? In order to reduce the study of gross anatomy in the dissection of cadavers to more reasonable proportions, I revised and rewrote a dissecting manual based on a practical anatomy book that I had myself used as a student originally written by my old Professor of Anatomy at St. Thomas's Hospital, F. G. Parsons, in collaboration with Professor W. Wright of the London Hospital. By the elimination of much unnecessary detail I was able to produce a single volume of comparatively slender dimensions that I hoped would replace the two- or three-volume manuals commonly used by medical students. I did not dare to make too drastic a reduction in the contents of my new manual, not to begin with at any rate, because I felt this would be regarded as too revolutionary a change by my anatomical contemporaries. But I had it in mind to make further reductions later on, if the book proved to be acceptable to them. However, though two editions appeared (in 1946 and 1949), the book was not a success and it subsequently went out of print. The reviews were polite but not enthusiastic, the main complaint being that too much detail had been eliminated and a few of the illustrations were too diagrammatic (though, in fact, these were intended to be diagrammatic for purposes of clarity). And now, as I write, the pendulum of the anatomical curriculum has swung much further than I had myself intended, and practical dissecting manuals have been replaced by skimpy paperback notebooks with the most meagre of directions for the procedure of dissection to guide the perplexed student, and the most schematic of line diagrams to indicate to him what is what. In the introduction to my book I wrote 'that the medical student's knowledge of topographical anatomy at the end of his preclinical course ought to be adequate for the following purposes—to provide a basis for an intellectual appreciation of the morphological principles which determine and influence the organization of the living body; to interpret in terms of structural organization the normal physiology of the human body (and therefore to anticipate the probable results of interference with normal structure and structural relationships); to recognize the anatomical basis of clinical signs and symptoms of disorder due to injury or disease; to understand the anatomical factors involved in the development of pathological processes and the possible complications that may arise therefrom; and to employ competently all the ordinary methods of examination and treatment (including minor surgery) which involve anatomical knowledge'. This seems to me to be a reasonable statement, and I have serious doubts whether the stringent emaciation of gross topographical anatomy in the preclinical curriculum of some universities that is now fashionable can possibly meet all the elementary requirements set forth therein. But pendulums, by their nature, do swing to and fro and, so far as the anatomical curriculum is concerned, it may well be that the pendulum of the anatomical curriculum will swing back again to assume a less extreme position.

This discursive and disjointed narrative of some of the activities and incidents that I experienced at Oxford may give the false impression that my time was entirely taken up with University duties of one sort or another. But during the twenty-eight years that I occupied the Chair of Anatomy I had many outside duties to attend to, such as examining medical students at other universities or giving special lectures, attending meetings of the Council of the Royal Society, the Medical Research Council, the Council of the British Association for the Advancement of Science, the Council of the Zoological Society, and the Court of the Salters' Company (a City Company of which my ancestors had been members of the livery for over two hundred years and which now devotes the bulk of its funds to the promotion of research in industrial chemistry), and other meetings of various kinds. The years were also interspersed from time to time with visits to universities abroad, in Europe, America, South Africa, Australia and New Zealand, in the course of which I gave lectures and very quickly learnt to appreciate the generous hospitality that I received from my hosts in many parts of the world. There were also occasional expeditions to central and southern Africa to examine sites, in caves or river gravels and other sedimentary deposits, where remains of early man and his stone implements had been discovered by local archaeologists. Then, during the last two years preceding my retirement, my attention came to be concentrated intensively on the rebuilding and extension of the Department of Anatomy, as the result of which its total accommodation was almost trebled. I confess to having felt a sense of pride in this achievement, for the building when finally completed equalled, and in some ways surpassed, in its design and equipment any of the equivalent departments that I had seen either in this country or abroad. But it was an achievement that owed its success to the co-operation and advice I continually received from many members of my staff—the teaching and research staff as well as the technical staff of laboratories, the departmental workshop, the photographic unit, and so forth. Of these my greatest debt was to Dr. Graham Weddell, who showed a remarkable insight into all the intricacies of what may be called the engineering problems of laboratory planning. It was due to his perspicacity that a number of interesting innovations were introduced into the design of the new department, and that difficulties of space and equipment were overcome that might otherwise have been unforeseen.

I had drawn up preliminary plans for a new Department of Anatomy as far back as 1938, but these had of course to be put aside at the outbreak of war in 1939. It was for me a particularly happy circumstance that my aspirations should finally come to be realized at the very end of my Oxford career.

CHAPTER 7

EXPLORING THE BRAIN

ANYONE who has seen a fresh human brain, or for that matter the brain of a good-sized animal such as a sheep, will know that to superficial inspection it consists of a soft pulpy substance, and he may well be led to wonder how such an apparently structureless mass can serve all the diverse functions that are attributed to it. Similar doubts were expressed over three hundred years ago by Thomas Sydenham, who was one of the notable worthies of Magdalen Hall, which in the nineteenth century became Hertford College. Sydenham was evidently not very enthusiatic about the contributions that the study of the anatomy of the brain could be expected to make towards the advancement of clinical diagnosis and treatment—in fact, he spoke of anatomical investigations with a good deal of disparagement. Referring to the brain he wrote that it 'is the source of sense and motion. It is the storehouse of thought and memory as well. Yet no diligent contemplation of its structure will tell us how coarse a substance (a mere pulp, and that not over nicely-wrought), should subserve so noble an end. No-one, either, can determine, from the nature and structure of its parts, whether this or that faculty would be exerted.' And even in quite recent years a psychologist has remarked that, so far as higher mental activities and their functional disturbances were concerned, the anatomist and physiologist could offer no assistance to their understanding— the skull might just as well be filled with cotton wool. Such pessimistic meanderings find no justification today; during the last twenty years or more the elucidation of cerebral functions has proceeded with ever increasing acceleration, not only in respect of Sydenham's 'sense and motion', but also in respect of the essential part played by certain elements of the brain in the much more complex faculties of the mind, including those that involve emotional experiences and the disorders to which they may be subjected in psychopathic conditions. It was as a direct result of these anatomical and physiological studies that there developed a form of treatment commonly known as 'psychosurgery' in which the connexions of limited regions of the brain were deliberately interrupted in order to correct otherwise intractable emotional aberrations.

If the pulpy substance of a fresh brain is sliced open, it is immediately apparent that it is by no means homogeneous even in its gross structure. For one thing, it is seen to be made up of white matter and grey matter. The white matter is white because it is composed of densely packed bundles of microscopically small nerve fibres each of which is ensheathed by a fine coat of fatty tissue. The grey matter is grey because it is largely composed of clusters or layers of nerve cells, and a large proportion of the nerve fibres that it also contains are not insulated by fatty sheaths—they are, so to speak, naked. The grey matter on the surface of the main part of the brain, the cerebral hemisphere, is thrown into a complicated pattern of convoluted folds; this is the cerebral cortex. Buried in the depths of the brain are other masses of grey matter, some of which are predominantly sensory in function and directly or indirectly receive incoming messages from the various special sense organs, from a diversity of sensory spots densely sprinkled over the whole area of the skin, from muscles and joints, from visceral organs, and so forth. Of these sensory receiving stations the most conspicuous is a large oval mass of grey matter called the thalamus, buried in the middle of the brain. Other clumps of grey matter are directly or indirectly concerned with motor functions; by their activity are determined the intensity and sequence of contraction of the numerous muscles of the body required for movements of one sort or another. Superimposed functionally over these lower-level centres of the brain that are implicated in the reception of sensory information and in control of muscular mechanisms is the cerebral cortex. In man and the higher mammals (particularly the higher Primates such as man, apes and monkeys), sensory messages in general must be relayed to sensory receiving areas of the cortex (for the most part from the thalamus) before they can be first analysed and finally synthesized in such a way as to present to the brain the ever-changing sensory pictures of the external and internal environment. And it is upon the cerebral cortex that mainly depends the mysterious phenomenon whereby sensory messages conducted along series of nerve fibres in the form of swiftly travelling electrical changes are transmuted into conscious experiences. There are also emissive motor areas of the cerebral cortex whose function it is to integrate and co-ordinate the activities of various lower motor centres in order to effect harmonious movements involving muscles in different parts of the body. But, of course, the situation is far more complicated than this. For one thing, the sensory and motor areas of the cerebral cortex are themselves intimately interlinked through the so-called 'association areas' of the cortex, and the latter are again interconnected anatomically and functionally among themselves. Thus, in spite of the fact that a number of different functional regions of the brain can be delineated, in the normal individual the brain together with the rest of the nervous system always acts as a whole, and the resultant of any activity of this system depends on very much more than just the sum of the activities of its several parts.

The association areas of the cortex become more obtrusive in the larger brains of the more advanced types of mammal, related to an increasingly greater complexity of behavioural reactions. Among the smaller lemurs, for example, and also in the small brain of the primitive tree-shrews, they are quite limited in extent as compared with those cortical areas primarily concerned with the reception of sensory messages from the eye, the ear, the skin and so forth. In the more advanced lemurs the association areas have become further expanded and still more so in monkeys and apes, and they attain their greatest extent in the human brain. Thus, if you examine the brains in this ascending scale of living Primates you find a progressive development of the association areas that evidently parallels the course of evolution of the Primate brain in past ages.

Fundamentally, the incessant interaction of different parts of the nervous system that occurs during waking life, and even during natural sleep in the regulation of automatic functions of the body, is mediated by the messages, or nerve impulses as they are called, which sweep with almost incredible velocity along nerve fibres to and from nerve cells. It is the task of the anatomist to follow the course of those nerve fibres that link up one part of the nervous system with another, and in this way to find clues regarding the functional significance of the messages and of the groups of nerve cells to or from which they are conveyed. My own interest in the structure and functions of the brain was first aroused when I was studying the anatomy of two little animals, the tree-shrew and the tarsier, specimens of which (as I have already mentioned) I had collected on my jungle expeditions in Borneo and which I brought back to England with me. In both these creatures the eyes are highly developed to an advanced degree, and the nervous pathways connecting the sensitive membrane of the eye, the retina, with the lower visual centres of the brain, and ultimately with the visual area of the cerebral cortex, are abundant and well-defined. To a very limited extent I could follow these pathways with the use of a dissecting microscope, but such a method can do no more than give provisional results that need to be confirmed by much more exacting experimental studies. Nerve fibres have to be followed individually, and individual nerve fibres can only be discerned under the high magnifications of a microscope. Even so, however, the precise origin, course and termination of individual fibres must still be ultimately determined with precision by the use of experimental methods or by the minute study of pathological lesions in patients who have died of injuries or disease of some part of the nervous system.

If a very thin section of a part of the brain is examined with a microscope, the profusion of nerve fibres running in all directions immediately strikes the eye. The appearance is one of an inextricable tangle of undergrowth of a dense jungle, the main denizens of the jungle being the nerve cells either scattered diffusely, or grouped into clumps or stratified layers. The nerve fibres are all formed as elongated outgrowths of cells—some relatively short expansions, others travelling as exceedingly fine threads for considerable distances. A fibre may end by making a contact with another nerve cell (the junctional contact is called a 'synapse'), so that messages are passed from cell to cell in a series of relays over many different regions of the brain and spinal cord. Those motor fibres that issue from the central nervous system terminate in single muscle fibres or gland cells each of microscopic dimensions— they convey messages that signal to muscles or glands the necessary requirements for co-ordinated muscular contractions and glandular activity.

In the higher Primates, and also to a lesser extent in the tree-shrews, a proportion of the nerve fibres from the eyes that run back over the base of the brain as the optic tracts end in a circumscribed mass of nerve cells in the thalamus called the 'geniculate body'. Now, it is an interesting fact that in most of the higher Primates this body consists of six compact layers of nerve cells, and it had been claimed by a Swiss neurologist that in the geniculate body of each side optic tract fibres from one eye (and of course the impulses that they carry) terminate exclusively in three of these layers, and those from the other eye in the other three layers. It seemed odd to me that this important observation had not attracted the attention that it really deserved. I resolved, therefore, to follow it up by further studies, and this I did initially by the microscopical examination of the brain of a monkey that had died at the London Zoo some years after it had lost one eye in fighting with one of its companions, and also the brain of a human patient who had died two years after the removal of one eye for glaucoma. The results of these studies were quite clear-cut; they fully confirmed the observation that optic fibres from the eye of the same side and those from the opposite side (that is to say, uncrossed and crossed fibres) undergo complete segregation in the geniculate body so as to end separately each in a set of three layers of nerve cells. This illustrates a curious and so far a quite mysterious principle in the organization of the pathways of the nervous system. The optic nerves travel back from the eyes conveying messages from the retina, and when they enter the brain-case they unite at the base of the brain to form a bridge, or chiasma. In the latter some of the fibres from each eye cross over to the optic tract of the opposite side, while others remain uncrossed and continue their journey back in the optic tract of the same side. In other words, each optic tract contains a mixture of crossed and uncrossed optic fibres. But my further experimental studies showed that the crossed and uncrossed fibres are completely, and apparently indiscriminately, mixed up in the optic tract—it is only when the latter actually reaches the geniculate body that they become, as it were, unshuffled and sharply segregated so that they are brought to their termination in different layers of cells. All the cells of the geniculate body send *their* fibres to that part of the cerebral cortex that is concerned with visual perception—the visual cortex as it is called; it may be said, therefore, that the geniculate body is a relay station through which the messages conveyed by the fibres of the optic nerve are relayed to the higher functional levels of the cerebral cortex, eventually there to give rise to conscious visual sensations. But the geniculate body is more than a relay station, it is also, and more important-ly, a sorting station where nerve fibres from the retina are sorted out into different categories having different functional significance. This 'sorting principle' in the analysis of sensory messages from sense organs to the brain has proved to be a very important factor in the organization of the nervous system—indeed, it seems to be a general phenomenon that underlies all our powers of discrimination in sensory perception, and the mechanism whereby the sorting is achieved so far remains entirely inexplicable. Let me give another simple example of this sorting principle. My colleague, Dr G. M. Weddell, who was interested in the patterns of nerve supply to the skin, found that the sensory nerve fibres from different local areas of a rabbit's ear become shuffled together in an apparently random disarrangement in the main sensory nerve that leaves the ear on its way to the spinal cord. But when this nerve actually reaches the spinal cord the fibres become unshuffled again so that each little constituent bundle is once more exclusively made up of fibres that originally came from one small local skin area of the ear. Of course, it is only by a sorting mechanism of this kind that we are able, by means of messages that reach the brain, to localize in our mind the exact position where we are touched by a fine wisp of cotton wool (even when our eyes are shut).

A much more striking demonstration of the sorting and segregation of sensory nerve fibres on their way to sensory centres in the brain was made by an American anatomist. He cut through the optic tract of newts and tadpoles. The fibres of the tract underwent regeneration and grew back once more to the brain. But at the site of the scar where the cut had been made the fibres were seen to be intertwisted in an apparently inextricable tangle. Yet when they reached their termination in the brain they had become unravelled again so that each small group of fibres eventually came to make contact with the nerve cells with which they had originally been connected. And the same thing happened if, after cutting through the optic tract, the eye was rotated 180° from its normal position; in this case experimental observations showed that the animal was viewing the world upside-down! Some other American scientists, studying the visual pathways in frogs by recording the electrical activity of single nerve fibres, found that in the optic nerve the constituent fibres follow sinuous paths, constantly shifting their relative position so that two neighbouring fibres in the nerve 'may come from as widely separated retinal areas as possible'—but the fibres 'congregate again at their terminals, not only according to their points of origin (in the retina) but also according to their functions'. How on earth do nerve fibres (and not only sensory nerve fibres but also motor fibres that innervate muscles) get sorted out in this fashion in accordance with their functional significance and with their sites of origin or their destination? We just do not know—it remains one of the most fundamental mysteries of the organization of the brain, and until this mystery has been resolved we shall remain very far from understanding how the brain works, and, still more, how conscious processes of discriminatory sensory perception and motor control are mediated by the brain.

As I have indicated, the main task of the anatomist in the study of the nervous system is to trace the origin, course and termination of bundles of nerve fibres linking sense organs with the brain and spinal cord, or conveying motor signals to muscles and glands, or relaying messages from one group of nerve cells to another in the central nervous system. The object of such investigations is to throw light on the functional import of the complexity of elements, fibre pathways and clumps of nerve cells and so forth, that compose the essential structure of the nervous system. How is this task approached? You can cut continuous sequences of extremely thin sections through the whole brain (cutting them with an apparatus called a microtome), and after staining them with different kinds of dyes examine them under a microscope. But this does not carry you very far because you can never be exactly certain where a nerve fibre seen in such sections, or a group of nerve fibres, has its origin or its termination. It is in order to reach certainty on these points that it is necessary to resort to experimental material—either 'natural' experiments in which a focal lesion of the brain or spinal cord has been made as the result of injury or disease (with subsequent death of the patient), or animal experiments in which small circumscribed lesions have been produced under suitable anaesthesia, and the brain later studied under the microscope.

In principle, the basis of such experimental studies is simple of explanation, though they involve difficult techniques that need to be applied with the greatest care, and the results require a very critical examination. If a group of nerve cells is destroyed, then the nerve fibres to which they give rise undergo a rapid degeneration. Similarly, if nerve fibres are interrupted, those that are cut off from their cells of origin also degenerate. The degenerating fibres can be detected under the microscope by special methods of staining, and in this way they can be distinguished from normal nerve fibres and traced to their actual termination whether (as in the brain or spinal cord) they end by making contact with other nerve cells, or, in the case of peripheral nerves, they make terminal connexions with muscle fibres or gland cells. And with the development of the very high-power resolution of electron microscopy, the exact position of degenerating nerve fibre terminals where they make contact with other cells can be defined with the greatest precision. It is also the case that if a bundle of nerve fibres is cut through, then the cells from which they have their origin usually undergo a process of degeneration that can be recognized by the application of other kinds of staining methods. Thus, if it is required to know where a bundle of nerve fibres comes from and where it goes to, this information can be obtained by following under the microscope the course and termination of the degenerating nerve fibres that have been cut off from their nerve cells, and also searching through the brain and spinal cord for the affected nerve cells (from which they originate) that have undergone the usual process of what is called 'retro-grade degeneration'. It is by such methods that nerve fibres conveying messages from all the various sense organs have been traced to lower-level centres in the central nervous system, and fibres conveying motor messages to activate muscles or glands have been traced from their primary origins in the brain or spinal cord.

It was by the study of retrograde degeneration that in the earlier days of my research work I traced out many of the pathways along which various clumps of nerve cells in the thalamus relay the sensory messages that they receive to differ-ent areas of the cerebral cortex, these areas being for the most part distinguished by differences in their microscopical appearance and arranged in a sort of mosaic patchwork over the cortex. This reference to the thalamus reminds me of an amusing incident in connexion with my election to the Chair of Anatomy at Oxford. The word 'thalamus', applied by anatomists of old to the main sensory mass of grey matter in the middle of the brain, means an inner chamber or a couch, and more specifically a bridal couch. Some of the members of the electoral committee were not anatomists or even scientists, and when one of the anatomical members supported my claims for the appointment by saying that I had 'put in some very good work on the thalamus' this naturally aroused a good deal of merriment.

There are still other means for the localization of fibre tracts and groups of nerve cells that have their specific functions. For example, there is a compact bundle of nerve fibres running down the length of the spinal cord called the 'pyramidal tract'. If this is interrupted unilaterally by injury or disease, partial or complete paralysis of voluntary movements of the limbs of one side occurs. Local lesions in certain parts of the brain produce the same effect. And there is a vertical strip of grey matter in the cerebral cortex (commonly called the 'motor cortex') which contains the nerve cells from which many of the fibres of the pyramidal tract arise. It is of particular interest that these cells are arranged in serial order from above downwards, so that those above are involved in the control of the movements of the leg, those in the middle the movements of the arm, and those below the movements of the face, lips and tongue, Behind the motor cortex is another vertical strip of grey matter, the general sensory cortex, and here again, it has been possible to show that certain localized bundles of nerve fibres carrying sensory messages up the spinal cord transmit these messages through relay stations so that different parts of the body are, so to speak, represented in the same sort of serial order.

There is yet another method of tracking the connexions between different elements of the central nervous system, and between these and the various sense organs. This is commonly called the electro-physiological method, but it might equally well be called the electro-anatomical method. In principle it depends on the stimulation (by electrical or chemical excitants) of sense organs, or nerve cells, or fibre tracts, and recording the resultant electrical activity engendered at their terminal stations. This is a very precise method and, by using it as complementary to the other methods that I have briefly mentioned, the interconnexions of the nervous system have been mapped out in great detail with considerable accuracy. One of the surprising results of all these studies has been the demonstration that in the brain there is a very fine degree of functional localization in its different parts—surprising because there was at one time a good deal of animated controversy on this particular problem. There were those who steadfastly opposed the idea of such a degree of functional localization in the brain—the latter, they maintained, always acted 'as a whole'. Of course, in a sense, they were right. But they did not realize that in order to act as a whole the brain must first be concerned with the analysis of incoming messages and the separate assortment of outgoing messages before all these can be synthesized to permit total patterns of sensations, or closely co-ordinated movements involving the concerted and nicely timed contraction of a number of different muscles. In other words, the functions of the central nervous system are both analytic and synthetic, but synthesis must necessarily be preceded by analysis. At the hinder extremity of the convoluted cerebrum is the patch of grey cortex, the visual cortex, that receives messages from the retina of the eye, and here each local area of the retina is projected on to a correspondingly local area of the cortex so that a small injury to the latter may lead to a circumscribed patch of blindness in the field of vision. In the same way, in the auditory cortex (in the temporal region of the cerebrum) sounds of different pitch reach the cortex in serial order as a sort of spatial reproduction of the tonic scale. The resultants of all such analytical procedures as these are flashed along interconnecting fibres to the association areas of the cerebral cortex and here are brought into the most intimate relationship with each other, and with innumerable other messages reaching the brain from sense organs in all other parts of the body. Thus the brain is ultimately presented with a *total* pattern of sensory inflow providing information of all that is going on outside the body as well as of changes that at the same time may be occurring inside the body. Furthermore, all this information about contemporary events is brought into relationship with stored information derived from the past events, that is to say, with what we call 'memory'. It is in this way that, through the brain, an individual can, consciously or unconsciously, make all the appropriate adjustments necessary to deal with new situations as they arise by regulating the activity of muscles, glands, and so forth.

From what I have said, it will be agreed that the tracking of all the complex interconnexions of the brain has a supreme importance for understanding just how the nervous system works in determining our behaviour under varying circumstances. This work of tracking is an exciting adventure in itself, but it is also quite an arduous adventure because of all the technical difficulties involved. The value of the clinical application of the knowledge thus acquired for the recognition and treatment of injury or disease of the nervous system can hardly be overestimated, and it is now possible in many cases to localize with precision the site of the damage by noting the functional defects that result from it. For example a small tumour pressing on the upper end of the motor cortex may give rise to a paralysis of some of the movements of one leg. A small circumscribed injury to the visual cortex may be precisely localized by charting the field of vision and outlining a circumscribed patch of blindness on a special chart used for this purpose. Lesions involving certain local regions of some of the association areas of the cerebral cortex may result in curious defects of speech and the understanding of language whether spoken or written. Once the precise area of damage to the brain has been thus defined, the possibility of dealing with the damage by surgical means can be considered. In such a way, the neurological anatomist can add his contribution to the welfare of mankind.

There are two interesting features of the interconnexions of different parts of the nervous system that deserve mention. One is that messages sweeping along nerve fibres and conveying signals to nerve cells are not always concerned with exciting these cells into activity; some (called inhibiting fibres) have a 'damping down' effect, so that they prevent, instead of initiating, activity. This is a most important function, for in the nervous system (as indeed in all other systems of the body) it is necessary to have a mechanism that can control and regulate behavioural reactions by inhibiting those activities that are not required and thus avoiding a sort of chaotic disorder. For example, the motor fibres of the pyramidal tract in the spinal cord eventually make contact with nerve cells in different levels of the cord whose fibres pass out in the peripheral nerves to various muscles. But these nerve cells must not all be thrown into action; in some movements of the limbs certain muscles are required to contract vigorously, but others are required to relax and remain inactive. The latter are prevented from a forcible contraction by inhibiting messages that reach the motor nerve cells from which they receive their innervation. Thus, when you bend your elbow, you do so by contracting your biceps muscle that lies in the front of the arm; but at the same time the triceps muscle that lies on the back of the arm and is used for straightening the arm must relax, and this it does by the inhibition of the appropriate motor nerve cells in the spinal cord. This is a very simple example of the function of inhibiting nerve fibres. In the whole of the nervous system they play a continuous role so that the resultant of any activity of the brain is determined by a nicely balanced combination of excitation and inhibition. Innumerable nerve cells are stimulated to action, but at the same instant, in order to achieve a precision of co-ordination, innumerable cells are damped down. It is like playing an organ of incredible complexity, continually pulling out and pushing in multitudes of stops to produce the harmonious cadences of a musical theme.

The other feature of nervous organization which is of the highest importance for the understanding of perceptual processes is this. Every sensory pathway through which information of the outside world is conveyed to the brain is associated with a system of outgoing, or centrifugal, nerve fibres that control and modify the sensory input. For example, centrifugal nerve fibres from the brain pass out along the optic tract to reach the retina where they make contact with sensory cells receiving visual stimuli engendered by light rays that are focussed on them through the lens of the eye. This means that the way in which the retinal cells react to visual stimuli, or indeed whether they react at all, can depend on outgoing messages from the brain. Hence patterns of light and colour that may exist externally in the field of vision are not necessarily reproduced with identical equivalence at what we may call the 'conscious levels' of the brain. This general principle of nervous organization—that is, the control and regulation of incoming messages from the outside world by outgoing messages from the brain itself, is applicable to all parts of the nervous system. Centrifugal fibres pass out to the sensory cells receiving odoriferous messages from the nose, to the sensory cells of the ear that respond to vibrations which we interpret as sounds, to the sensory corpuscles scattered over the surface of the skin that respond to touch, changes of temperature, or noxious agents that give rise to a feeling of pain. And in the brain itself sensory messages from lower functional levels are monitored by messages running in the reverse direction from higher functional levels. Obviously, all these reciprocal connexions have a profound significance for the study of perceptual phenomena because they determine that what we ultimately experience as a conscious sensation is not solely dependent on external stimuli alone; the effects of the latter may be variably conditioned by intrinsic activities emanating from the brain itself. In other words, altogether apart from the initial selection and fractionation of sensory messages dependent on limitations in the construction of our sense organs and the sensory receiving centres in the brain, there is opportunity for still further selective control of these messages by a 'censorship' imposed along outgoing pathways from different functional levels of the brain. It may be inferred, therefore, that the sensory material which ultimately reaches conciousness may be limited and fractionated to a degree that is hardly realizable. How far, in fact, can the conscious perceptions of each one of us reflect, or reproduce, all the patterned details of external reality? We just do not know.

It is in the upper part of the cerebrum that most of the important receiving mechanisms of the brain are situated, through which sensory messages are enabled to give rise to conscious perceptions. It is in this part of the brain, also, that lie the motor cortex and other nerve cell stations that are concerned with the initiation and control of muscular activities. Broadly speaking, then, much of this region of the brain is concerned with adjustments to changes in the external environment—the outside world. Right at the base of the brain, and therefore more difficult of access either for surgical treatment of patients or for experimental study of animals, are masses of grey matter consisting of numerous conglomerations of nerve cells which are concerned more with the internal environment—the inside world of the self.

It is only in comparatively recent years that the functional significance of various parts of this 'basal brain' has begun to be recognized, and this has been the combined result of intensive studies by anatomical and physiological methods, as well as by clinical observations. In one part of it are nerve cells that play a role in the temperature regulation of the body; in another part are groups of cells that help to govern the rate and intensity of the heart beat, or the movements of the digestive tract, or send nerve fibres down to end in the pituitary gland and mediate the secretory activities of this supremely important organ (supremely important because it dominates and controls the hormonal activities of various glands of internal secretion on which we depend for the continuing normal duties of many of our body functions). Another localized group of cells at the base of the brain has an astonishing effect on the appetite; if it is destroyed experimentally in a rat the animal develops a curious condition known as hyperphagia which manifests itself in such an insatiable appetite that it eats and eats to a most ungainly obesity. But apart from these unitary activities of various parts of the basal brain, injuries to the latter may lead to remarkable disturbances of emotional reactions—destruction of one complex of nerve cells may change an aggressive and untameable animal into a placid and docile one; destruction of another complex may have the opposite effect, producing rage reactions in animals that were previously tame and tranquil in their behaviour. And the same kind of changes in temperament and emotional reactions have been observed in human patients who have suffered injury to these parts of the brain. How can such phenomena be explained? The basal brain is clearly a very primitive part of the cerebrum concerned with, and regulating, what are called the vegetative functions of the body, that is to say, metabolic activities involving visceral and glandular mechanisms. By contrast, the main part of the convoluted cerebral cortex provides the neurological basis for the cognitive aspect of mental experience, the analysis and understanding of discrete events taking place in the outer world of events. But the two are interconnected by various nerve pathways. Thus, many of the vegetative activities of the basal brain are projected on to the cerebral cortex, particularly on those areas that form the frontal lobes of the brain. Conversely, descending pathways from the frontal lobes pass directly or indirectly to the basal brain, and it is seemingly through these that the frontal areas of the cortex can control and modify those regions of the basal brain that are involved in emotional reactions. All this has been made abundantly clear in the 'psychosurgical' operations that were at one time the fashionable treatment of disturbed mental conditions such as acute anxiety neurosis—operations that were called leucotomy. The idea of these operations was to sever the nerve pathways linking the frontal lobe with the basal brain. The results were sometimes very dramatic; the patient (at any rate for a time) lost his anxieties and became placid and easy-going. But often he became too easy-going and reckless, for he no longer displayed the normal inhibitions that are needed to maintain correct behaviour in a social group—he might become garrulously happy, inconsiderate towards his fellow-beings, and unable or unwilling to practise foresight in the planning activities of day-to-day routine. In fact, though he might appear to be much happier in a 'happy-go-lucky' sort of way, he might become an intolerable nuisance to his family and friends. The original crude operations of leucotomy became later replaced by more refined and local operations involving the destruction of only quite small areas of the cerebral cortex, but even these are now tending (at least in some cases) to be replaced by non-surgical methods of treatment, chemotherapy for instance, that are effective without awkward side-effects.

These interconnexions between the analytical mechanisms of the cerebral cortex and the primitive mass-reacting centres of the basal brain do not cover the whole story of brain and mental activity. By no means. They provide some of the anatomical basis in explanation of the fact that we can become consciously aware of our emotional impulses and at the same time learn to keep them under control. But there are other structures in the brain that also appear to play an important part in the total integration of its activities. One of these is a curious strip of cortical grey matter which insinuates itself into the wall of the ventricular cavity of the brain (for the brain is really hollow), and which becomes exposed on dissection as an elongated and curved eminence in the ventricular wall. This was called by the ancients the 'hippocampus' because of its fanciful resemblance to that unlikely-looking fish, the sea-horse (or, more probably, the anatomist who first coined this name about 400 years ago was thinking of the dolphin). The hippocampus has for many years been a puzzle to students of the brain; it is a constant component of the brain from the highest to the lowest vertebrates, and for long had been thought to be entirely concerned with the reception and interpretation of smell messages from the nose. But it is quite large in the human brain, and in man the sense of smell is but poorly developed. Experimental studies by myself and some of my colleagues failed to confirm the supposition that it is exclusively or even mainly, concerned with smell sensations, and yet, just because it is so universally present in vertebrates of all kinds, it must, we supposed, play a very fundamental part in cerebral activities. Hence, its anatomical connexions with other parts of the brain have been the subject of intensive investigations by numerous neuro-anatomists, in my own department particularly by my friends Tom Powell and Max Cowan and their collaborators. It now appears that the hippocampus receives, directly or indirectly, sensory messages of every possible kind from other parts of the brain. But what does it do with all this information that it acquires? Evidently it transmits it back to certain areas of the cerebral cortex again, for it sends off a compact bundle of nerve fibres that descend to the basal brain, from which they are relayed up to a group of nerve cells in the thalamus, and from this group another relay of fibres is despatched to a strip of cortex on the inner surface of each cerebral hemisphere. Thus it seems that the hippocampus is part of a 'feed-back' mechanism through which the activity of the cerebral cortex as a whole can be continually modulated in a positive or negative fashion. However, little is still certainly known about the significance of this circuit for the control of behaviour. What is certainly known is that if the hippocampus with its immediately adjacent region is destroyed either experimentally in animals, or by injury in human patients, the ability to remember anything is almost completely abolished. This is particularly the case with recent events—the memory of events even after so short an interval as two or three minutes is obliterated. Curiously enough, in certain cases (in human patients) some degree of memory for events long past may be retained, suggesting that the hippocampus and its neighbouring structures are concerned rather with the *initial* stages of memory storage in the brain, and that this storage is eventually mediated by other parts of the cerebral cortex.

It may be of parenthetic interest to note that the hippocampus was originally called the hippocampus major, because in the back part of the ventricular cavity of the brain is another, smaller, eminence in the wall of the ventricle that was called the hippocampus minor. It is a structure of no functional importance at all, being merely caused by an indentation of the ventricular wall by an unusually deep fissure in the overlying convoluted cerebral cortex. Yet it played a very curious part in biological history when it became the centre of a dramatic controversy between the celebrated anatomists T. H. Huxley and Sir Richard Owen (at that time the Conservator of the Hunterian Museum in the Royal College of Surgeons) shortly after Darwin's *Origin of Species* was published. In retrospect it seems odd that so much emphasis was laid on this insignificant and unimportant structure, but Owen maintained that it was a unique feature of the human brain that quite sharply distinguished man from the apes, using this feature to support his claim that man should, in a zoological classification, be placed in a separate division of his own, 'Archencephala', completely distinct from all other divisions of mammals. But Huxley had no difficulty in confirming previous observations of some continental anatomists that the hippocampus minor is also present in the chimpanzee's brain, and, indeed, it is also to be found in the brain of other Primates. This controversy reached a climax in the historical debate between Huxley and the Bishop of Oxford at a meeting of the British Association held at Oxford in 1860, and the debate is still commemorated by a plaque fixed to the door of the room in the Oxford Museum where it took place. An amusing satirical reference to this controversy was made by Charles Kingsley in his story of *The Water Babies*, a story that is subtitled 'a fairy tale', as indeed it is, though much of it would be quite unintelligible to young children and some of it, because of topical allusions, even to adults today. The particular allusion referring to the hippocampus minor (of which Kingsley makes a nomenclatural joke) occurs in chapter four of his book, where the little girl Ellie is walking along the sea-shore with a caricatured professor. The professor, Kingsley writes, 'held very strange theories about a good many things. He had even got up once at the British Association, and declared that apes had hippopotamus majors in their brains just as men have. Which was a shocking thing to say; for, if it were so, what would become of the faith, hope, and charity of immortal millions? You may think that there are other more important differences between you and an ape, such as being able to speak, and make machines, and know right from wrong, and say your prayers, and other little matters of that kind; but that is a child's fancy, my dear. Nothing is to be depended on but the great hippopotamus test. If you have a hippopotamus major in your brain, you are no ape, though you had four hands, no feet, and were more apish than the apes of all aperies. But if a hippopotamus major is ever discovered in one single apes's brain, nothing will save your great-great-great-great-great-great-great-great-great-great-great-greater-greatest-grandmother from having been an ape too. No, my dear little man; always remember that the one true, certain, final, and all-important difference between you and an ape is, that you have a hippopotamus major in your brain, and it has none; and that, therefore, to discover one in its brain will be a very wrong and dangerous thing, at which everyone will be very much shocked, as we may suppose they were at the professor.'

I have remarked that what I have called the 'basal brain' contains nervous mechanisms that control and regulate visceral and glandular functions and that in some manner they are involved in emotional reactions and emotional experiences. It is evident also, from clinical observations following destructive injuries of certain regions of the basal brain, that these may lead to profound changes in conscious attitudes, and even in the essence of consciousness itself. Certainly, through its intimate connexions with the hippocampus and related parts of the cerebral cortex it plays a significant role in the conscious recall of past experiences. Such observations naturally raise the intriguing problem of the relation of the purely neural activities of the brain to purely mental processes, that is to say, to the phenomenon of conscious awareness. There are those who would attribute some form of elementary awareness to all living organisms, from the highest to the lowest, and there are extremists who would extend this concept even to non-living matter. There are also philosophers who seem to deride the idea that consciousness is a distinct entity to be contrasted with purely physiological activities of the body and refer to it as the 'ghost in the machine'. I find it impossible to follow verbal peregrinations in such philosophical meanderings. To me consciousness *is* a distinct entity, even though my monistic attitude to existence compels me to suppose that in some mysterious way it is ultimately a coalescent extension of physiological activities mediated by the brain and other organs of the body. The only thing of which I am entirely certain is that I have a conscious awareness of myself and that I have conscious sensations that appear to reflect, perhaps only to a limited extent, a presumed reality of the external world. All else is inference based on these fundamental experiences. Descartes' well-known aphorism 'Cogito, ergo sum' still seems to me to be basically true in spite of the fact that it has been criticized as semantically obscure. There is evidently a concomitance of some sort between mind and matter and much has lately been written and discussed on this vital problem without very conclusive results. It is indeed, at any rate to my way of thinking, extremely difficult to conceive how electrical impulses passing along nerve fibres and exciting nerve cells to action or inactivating them can possibly be transmuted into a conscious experience. And yet the advent of the phenomenon of conscious awareness in the evolutionary process must presumably have a utilitarian value of some sort, and this assumption naturally raises the perennial question of free will —does it exist, or is it nothing more than a phantasm of the imagination? The President of the Royal Society in 1959, Sir Cyril Hinshelwood (at that time Professor of Physical Chemistry at Oxford), gave a memorable anniversary address in which he made reference to this problem. 'Of the concomitance of consciousness with brain processes there is no doubt, but concomitance does not mean identity. . . . Nor in a concomitance of A and B is it justifiable to assert that A is the cause of B without admitting the possibility of a reciprocal relation. In particular, if we assert that physical happenings in the brain can affect consciousness we must admit in principle that physical happenings in the brain may be consciously caused.' He also draws on the evolutionary principle of natural selection and remarks that 'if free will, moral feelings and other conscious elements are illusions superposed on a behaviouristic background, wherein can lie their selective advantage?'

Now, let us suppose that behaviour based on a decision from

a choice of one of several alternative courses of action is simply the resultant of physical processes involving nerve fibres and nerve cells in the brain; is there in fact any evidence that conscious deliberation can affect these processes? I think there is. In the psychoanalytical treatment of a mild obsessional neurosis (and I would stress the qualifying word 'mild' because there is serious doubt about the effectiveness of this method of treatment in severe cases), the patient's behavioural reaction to certain events may be entirely, and sometimes abruptly, changed from an abnormal compulsive reaction to a normal and rational reaction. Here, then, is an example where purely conscious processes can, it must be presumed, in some way alter or modify the neuronal circuits in the brain on which behavioural reactions depend. Such a phenomenon must surely be taken into account when the problem of free will is discussed.

Apart from general considerations of this kind, the physical substratum in the brain of consciousness has become more and more clearly defined in the last twenty years or so by experimental and clinical studies, though no amount of experimentation and clinical observation can decide whether consciousness is just mediated or influenced by physical activities of the nervous system, or whether it is an entity in its own right; whether, in fact, there is ultimately a duality of mind and matter even admitting that there may be an interaction between the two. But let us for the moment return to a brief consideration of certain anatomical features of the brain. The lowest functional levels of the brain comprise what is called the 'brain-stem', an upward continuation, in more elaborate and complex structure, of the spinal cord where this reaches the inside of the skull. Further up, the brain-stem plunges into the substance of cerebrum which, in the human brain, is largely made up of the convoluted cerebral cortex, the thalamus, the basal brain, as well as other masses of grey matter with all their interposed white matter of interweaving and interconnecting nerve fibres. For years past, students of the nervous system have tended to focus their attention on the well-defined and circumscribed bundles of nerve fibres each conveying messages of specific functional import, and on the well-defined and circumscribed groups of nerve cells receiving and relaying incoming messages that eventually give rise to conscious perceptions. But the destruction of any one of these sensory elements of the brain does not by itself abolish self-awareness, and this applies even to different sensory areas of the cerebral cortex. Of course, if the visual area of the cortex is completely destroyed, visual sensations are abolished—the patient is no longer conscious of messages sent back from the retina of the eye along the optic nerve. And a similar localized defect in the field of consciousness results from localized destruction of other sensory areas of the cortex. But conscious awareness of self remains undisturbed, and this is also the case if a single compact bundle of nerve fibres in the spinal cord or brain conveying sensory messages of a specific kind is interrupted. In other words, our specific sensations of vision, hearing, smell and so forth may be regarded as so many sensory experiences high-lighted on a background of a general awareness of self. This phenomenon is paralleled by the fact that discrete and circumscribed fibre tracts or groups of nerve cells in the brain stand out as 'high-lights' against a background of a diffuse matrix composed of scattered nerve cells and intricate networks of nerve fibres whose connexions and functions have been exceedingly difficult to analyse by anatomical and physiological methods. But in recent years their functional import has in some measure been elucidated, and the diffuse collections of cells and fibres has come to be included in the term 'reticular formation'.

The reticular formation of the central nervous system is perhaps the most primitive constituent of the brain—the essential matrix in which, during the evolutionary complexification of the nervous system, the more sharply defined fibre pathways and cell groupings subserving specific functions have, as it were, become gradually crystallized out as circumscribed anatomical elements. The reticular formation itself, however, remains and extends in continuity from the spinal cord, through the brain-stem, and into the substance of the thalamus, and by an intricate series of relays and interconnexions it has been shown to exert an influence on the activity of the cerebral cortex as a whole. Stimulation of some parts of the reticular formation in the brain-stem may enhance the activity of the cerebral cortex (as evidenced by its electrical responses), while stimulation of other parts may depress its activity. But the interesting thing is that, while interruption of the circumscribed pathways conveying messages related to discriminatory perceptions of visual images, sounds, pain and so forth does not affect conscious awareness, a complete blockage of the continuity of the reticular formation at any level in the brain by, say, a tumour or a massive haemorrhage in the brain, does lead to coma and unconsciousness. And if practically the whole cerebral cortex is destroyed (and not just localized areas), this also results in a loss of consciousness. So it looks as if the reticular formation is responsible, directly or indirectly, for maintaining and regulating the normal functions of the cerebral cortex as a whole. At any rate, the formation has come to be regarded as the 'stuff of consciousness' in the brain, and to it has been given the all-inclusive term—the centrencephalic system. The anatomical exploration of this system, as well as of the basal brain, the hippocampus and related structures, has been excessively tedious and time-consuming because of the technical difficulties that have had to be overcome by patient research workers. But the results so far achieved have been considerable as well as important. Nevertheless it has to be recognized that the functional implications of these studies are still far more clear. In particular, the concepts of 'consciousness' and 'awareness' are open to a good deal of criticism in regard to their precise definition. It may indeed be true that some sort of 'awareness', however vague and rudimentary, is an attribute of all living organisms. And in ourselves the construction of the brain has become amplified and complexified to the extent that we are enabled to perceive changes in the world around us and in ourselves with a far sharper discrimination than is possible for lower animals.

The brain has been compared by some enthusiastic investigators with electronic computers, and it has even been suggested that the latter can 'think'. But surely this is no more than an anthropomorphism. Long before computers were invented, there were ingenious mechanical feed-back devices which could easily have given an impression of intelligent action to those not conversant with the cunning details of their construction. It may well be that the brain, at any rate at its higher levels as represented by the cerebral cortex, is comparable to a computer of quite incredible complexity. But maybe it is an intangible agency generated by conscious activity—the mind, or the psyche (whatever you like to call it)—that in some manner makes use of this organic computer as a sort of control system whereby we are enabled to adjust our behaviour by appropriate responses to the sequences of change continually occurring in our external and internal environment. On the other hand, this is not to deny that the purely physical activities of the brain and the phenomenon of consciousness, that at present appear to us to be quite disparate entities, may ultimately be shown to be compatible with a monistic interpretation of existence.

CHAPTER 8

THE ANTIQUITY OF MAN

IN my early youth my brothers and I visited Kent's Cavern at Torquay, a cavern that is really a labyrinth of caves and connecting passages the first excavations of which were made in the early part of the last century. We were naturally interested to see fossilized relics of extinct creatures such as cave-bears still embedded in the stalagmitic matrix that had once filled parts of the cavern. But what impressed me most at the time was a large boulder of stalagmite, about six feet high, underneath which had been found a flint implement made by prehistoric man. Stalagmite, like stalactites suspended from the roof of such a cave, is slowly formed by the dripping of water containing lime salts. The water evaporates, leaving the lime salts as a permanent residue. The rate of formation of the stalagmite on the boulder to which I have referred had been measured year by year with a micrometer, and, if my recollection is correct, it was estimated that it would take about 12,000 years to add an inch thickness of stalagmite over the boulder. Evidently, then, the flint implement must have been made very many thousands of years ago, This, I think, was the first occasion on which I came to realize the vast antiquity of prehistoric man. Of course, this method of estimating antiquity is not very reliable, for the rate of deposition of stalagmite may have varied a good deal over the past, depending on variations in rainfall and other factors; nevertheless, the antiquity of that implement, humanly contrived, must have been very great. When flint implements were first discovered in Kent's Cavern in about 1820, the natural inference that they carried the age of mankind far back beyond the limits prescribed by the biblical story of creation aroused very considerable opposition. Many theologians of the time were content to accept the earlier estimate of Archbishop Ussher (an estimate ingeniously based on a calculation of the genealogical sequence of the descendants of Adam and Eve recorded in the Bible) that the creation of the world took place in the year 4004 B.C. Dean Buckland, then Professor of Geology at Oxford, argued that the evidence from Kent's Cavern substantiated the biblical story of the Flood, that the remains of extinct animals found there were the remains of antediluvian creatures, and that the supposed human artefacts known at that time were secondarily introduced at a later date. It was not until an amateur French archaeologist, Boucher de Perthes, in 1838 discovered undoubted flint implements called 'hand-axes' in what were clearly very ancient gravel deposits in the valley of the Somme, and which he ascribed to the work of 'antediluvial' populations, that the great antiquity of man came to be accepted by scientists as definitely proven. Even then, however, there were still sceptics. Today we know for certain that the family of mankind had already started on its evolutionary career thousands, and even some millions, of years ago.

There are a number of technical methods now available for estimating the relative or absolute age of geological deposits and their contained fossils, and some of these methods give a high degree of accuracy. But for me the most penetrating realization of antiquity is not so easily conceived by numerical reference to so many thousands, or hundreds of thousands, of years, as by seeing or finding the actual fossilized relics of early types of man and other animals still lying undisturbed in deposits laid down when many parts of the earth were vastly different from what they are today. Once, when I was walking with Dr Desmond Clark (one of the foremost, and certainly the soundest, authority on African archaeology) along the top of the Zambezi gorge some miles below the

Victoria Falls, where the river had cut through about 400 feet thickness of dense basaltic rock, we picked up stone implements in river gravels at the top of the gorge which must have lain there since the time when the Zambezi was still running at that level. In other words, since the implements were made by prehistoric man, the river had cut its way to a depth of 400 feet as far back as the Victoria Falls some miles upstream. On another occasion I accompanied the East African archaeologist, Dr Louis Leakey, to what is now a hot desert near the southern boundary of Kenya, a place called Olorgesailie. Aeons ago it was not a desert, for this area was then occupied by a great lake and on the shores of the lake there flourished a palaeolithic community. For some reason or another, perhaps because the level of the lake suddenly rose and flooded sites of habitation, the members of the community were compelled hurriedly to abandon their home. But they left behind them the products of their industry—hundreds of large stone hand-axes and cleavers that now lie scattered in marvellous profusion over the desert surface. This unique site was found by Mrs Leakey in 1942, and it now remains as a veritable natural museum bearing witness to the activities of early man in East Africa.

Human antiquity, I think, is impressed just as strongly by the evidence of the astonishingly high degree of technical skill and ingenuity shown in the work of co-operative communities in ancient times. Earthworks such as long and round barrows, or the earthwork surrounding the remnants of stone circles at Avebury, or the high fort with series of peripheral ramparts at Maiden Castle in Dorset—all these bear witness to lively and active communities capable of immense constructional efforts several thousand years ago. Experiments by archaeologists using simple tools such as antler picks, crude shovels and other implements available to men of those days have led to the conclusion that the earthwork at Avebury could only have been completed if some two hundred men had laboured over a period of nine years. My own realization of the technical 'know-how' and of the acute insight of ancient populations of Britain somewhere about 3,500 years ago first dawned on me when I visited Stonehenge. Gazing at this prodigious monument I wondered at their ability to transport the blue stones (probably from South Wales by rafts or boats up the Bristol Channel and then overland), and the efforts required to drag the great sarsen stones of many tons weight from the Marlborough Downs twenty miles away to their present site. All this sheer physical effort must have occupied the energies of hundreds of men over many years. But, apart from these feats of strength and endurance, how amazingly accurate must have been their computations to be able to erect the stone circles in such a way as to fit in so precisely with the sunrise at the summer solstice! Once, standing on the Great Wall of China, my imagination momentarily conjured up a most vivid scene of the multitudes of men engaged in the construction of this remarkable monument of military engineering over 2,000 years ago. The wall is twenty feet high with a roadway fifteen feet wide at its top, and with a fortified tower every hundred yards or so. From the top you can see it twisting and turning its serpentine course over hills, along ridges and over valleys as it proceeds on its uninterrupted zig-zag way for a matter of eighteen hundred miles, and you see it fading into the bleak and rugged distance like some gigantic switchback. The wall was contrived with the purpose of keeping out the nomadic 'barbarians' from their periodic incursions into northern China, and, according to some accounts, it was built by the forced labour of many thousands of men (according to legend as many as 300,000) working under incredibly harsh conditions and suffering a terrible mortality rate by disease, starvation, exposure, exhaustion, or even deliberate butchery at the hands of cruel task-masters.

But such relics of early civilizations take us nowhere near

the beginnings of cultural skill in human prehistory. Creep your way down into the depths of some of the caves at Les Eyzies in the Dordogne region of France, as I did in 1930, and examine the polychrome mural paintings, and the carvings in bas relief, the work of men of the Old Stone Age. For paintings the artists used black manganese oxide and red and yellow ochre, durable pigments that still look surprisingly fresh. It is a thrilling experience to see these artistic representations of animals that lived in those days—life-like representations of horses, bisons, reindeer, cave-bear, cave-lion, mammoth and woolly rhinoceros. Their artistic merit is beyond doubt, and there is good evidence that some of them date back to about 15,000 years ago, others almost 30,000 years ago. The profusion of paintings suggest an art gallery, but sanctuary is a better term for they are to be found in the darker recesses of the caves and they could only have been made with the dim light of exceedingly primitive and crude oil lamps. Their purpose was clearly propitiatory for success in hunting, for most of the animals portrayed are those that provided food for palaeolithic man. And there are also representations of the female figure whose emphasis on sexual features makes it reasonably certain that they were associated with fertility rites. The artists responsible for these cave paintings were members of a community highly adept in the fabrication of beautifully made flint implements, of harpoons of antler, of bone awls and needles, and many other tools. It is evident, therefore, that they had already achieved at that time a very intricate and well developed material culture associated with quite an advanced social organization.

This mention of the cultural achievements brings me to the question of how the antiquity of palaeolithic man and his predecessors has been determined. There are two main methods of establishing the chronology of fossil man and other animals—relative dating and absolute dating. Relative dating can be determined by what are called stratigraphical levels. The principle is simple enough to understand, though in practice the method needs to be applied by skilled geologists. If a river overflows and spreads across its banks a thick layer of sediment sufficiently rapidly to bury under it the carcass of an animal, the bones of the latter may in course of time become preserved in a fossilized form. Further layers of silt may later be deposited one by one over the first in a series of stratifications. It is clear, then, that fossils found embedded in the deeper layers will be more ancient than those found in the more superficial layers. The same principle applies to the drippings of lime impregnated water on to the floor of caves, forming successive layers of stalagmite, or to mud, gravel and sand deposited in lakes and seas. Mud may become consolidated to form shale or slate, sand and gravel may become consolidated to form sandstone, or a sort of 'breccia'. In either case, this ensures a more complete and permanent preservation of the skeletons of animals that maybe lived thousands or even millions of years ago. If a fossil is found at the bottom of a great mass of stratified deposits, perhaps several hundred feet thick, obviously it must be of very considerable antiquity, and by observing the nature and thickness of the overlying strata it may be possible to make a very rough guess of its probable antiquity in terms of years. But such guesses are of precarious value. However, during the geological period when mankind was evolving, called the Pleistocene period, there were periodic climatic changes of considerable magnitude—cold and subtropical alternations in the northern and southern hemispheres, wet and dry alternations in tropical regions. The climatic environment can often be determined by the nature of the geological deposit, or by the kinds of fossilized animals and plants which they contain. During the latter half of the Pleistocene period there were at least four successive glaciations in northern Europe and America, as well as some minor ones. In England, for example, the glaciations extended over Scotland and the northern part of England, in one case even extending as far down as the river Thames. One can picture at these times great glaciers spreading down from the Arctic region, scooping out steep-sided valleys and lake basins, scraping and scratching the rocks over which they scoured their downward flow, and leaving behind (where they melted) the characteristic débris of what is called 'boulder-clay'. It is by reference to such features that the action of the long-past glaciers can still be recognized by geologists—or, for that matter, by any observant person who wanders over the countryside of Scotland and northern England. From various pieces of evidence, mutually confirmatory, it is reckoned that the first major glaciation of the Ice Age reached its climax 600,000 years ago, the second about 350,000 years, the third (and most severe) about 150,000 years, and the last about 50,000 years. Remains of prehistoric man have been found in deposits laid down in various of the glacial or interglacial series, and if it can be determined, as it sometimes can be, to which of these climatic oscillations the deposits may be referred, the relative antiquity of their contained fossils can also be determined.

The other noteworthy method of relative dating is called the fluorine method. It depends on the fact that when fossil bones lie in a porous soil they gradually take up the chemical element fluorine from percolating water and this becomes fixed in the bony tissue as a very stable compound called fluorapatite. Thus, the longer a bone remains embedded in the soil, the more fluorine will it contain, and of course the amount of fluorine can be estimated by chemical tests. But the amount of fluorine taken up in this way also depends on the concentration of the element in the soil and it therefore does not permit a comparison of the relative antiquity of fossilized bones from different deposits in which the fluorine content may vary widely. On the other hand, if, say, a human skull is found in a deposit side by side with bones of long extinct elephants and other animals known to have lived thousands of years ago, then the fluorine test is of the highest importance, for it can determine whether the skull became embedded contemporaneously with the animal bones, or whether it reached its position secondarily as the result of a subsequent interment. For example, there was a famous human skeleton found in gravel deposits at Galley Hill in the Thames valley which for many years was held to be of great antiquity until the negligible value of its fluorine content demonstrated that it was of comparatively recent origin. Again, it was the fluorine test, applied by my friend Dr Kenneth Oakley, that first drew attention to the anomaly of the infamous Piltdown Skull, later to be exposed as a most unscrupulous forgery the details of which are recounted in the next chapter.

Methods of absolute dating are of course much more satisfying than relative dating. One of these is the radio-carbon method. When we breathe, we take in small quantities of carbon dioxide, and an extremely minute proportion of the carbon is radioactive. Thus, during life radioactive carbon is assimilated into living tissues in a fixed amount, and this applies to all living organisms, whether animals or plants. But after the organism has died, the radioactive carbon undergoes a slow disintegration at a known rate uninfluenced by temperature, humidity or any other environmental change. In other words the proportion of radioactive carbon to ordinary carbon progressively diminishes in dead organic material in relation to its antiquity, and by estimating the proportions of the two the absolute age in terms of years can be calculated with fair accuracy. Unfortunately the method is not applicable to fossil remains much older than about 50,000 years because of technical difficulties in the analysis of the material. But it is by this method that the earlier artists of cave paintings are reckoned to have lived almost 30,000 years ago.

Another method is available for estimating the absolute antiquity of older fossil remains—the potassium-argon method. Natural potassium compounds in certain minerals, for example those found in volcanic ashes, contain a minute amount of radioactive potassium which in the course of a gradual decay disintegrates to form two elements, calcium and argon. It takes about 1,300 million years for the radioactive potassium to be reduced to half its original amount in this way, and, by estimating the amount of the radioactive element in relation to the products of its disintegration in appropriate minerals from a geological deposit, it is possible to calculate the antiquity of the latter (and therefore of any fossils that it may contain) over a period of millions of years. It is by this method that the Pleistocene period has been shown to have extended much further back in time than had previously been supposed —about three million years. Incidentally, we may note that by the same method the preceding geological period, the Pliocene, began about twelve million years ago, and the still earlier Miocene period about twenty-five million years ago.

Now let us return to prehistoric man. We have made mention of later palaeolithic communities that flourished towards the end of the Pleistocene period. They were succeeded, about 7,000 years ago, by neolithic peoples, who by this time had learned the art of making more efficient stone implements by grinding and polishing them into appropriate shapes with fine cutting edges (instead of just chipping them), and who built villages, made pottery, domesticated animals, cultivated cereals, and hunted with bows and arrows. This neolithic phase of cultural and social development first arose somewhere in the Middle East and did not reach Britain until about 2500 B.C. We know from their skeletal remains that in their physical characters they were quite similar to modern Europeans, that is to say, they were fully developed *Homo sapiens*. This raises the interesting question—how old is *Homo sapiens*? The later

CPE O

palaeolithic populations, like their neolithic successors, were also indistinguishable, at any rate in the details of skull and other parts of the skeleton, from modern man. But in Europe during the severities of the last glaciation, about 40,000 to 50,000 years ago, another type of humanity existed—Neanderthal man. He was a curious and seemingly primitive type, for he had a retreating forehead, heavy and massive brow ridges, large and protruding jaws with no chin eminence, and coarsely built limb bones. At one time this type of Neanderthal man was taken to be the direct ancestor of *Homo sapiens*, and he was given the name *Homo primigenius*. But we know now that he suddenly became extinct towards the end of the last major glaciation of the Ice Age and was replaced by men of modern type who probably invaded Europe from the Near East and, it is presumed, exterminated him. But we must go back still further in time.

During the last interglacial phase of the Ice Age between the third and fourth glaciations, about 100,000 years ago or so, the few human remains that have been found which can with reasonable certainty be dated to that time are those of individuals whose skulls are somewhat 'neanderthaloid' in appearance with strongly built brow ridges (though not so accentuated as those of later Neanderthal man), but in the shape of the skull as a whole they were hardly distinguishable from *Homo sapiens*. Indeed, there seems no good reason for excluding them from this species. It is customary now to refer to them as 'generalized neanderthaloids' and in this way to distinguish them from the extreme or specialized neanderthaloids who occupied Europe during the last major glaciation. Although the fossil evidence is still rather meagre, it does suggest that towards the latter part of the last interglacial period populations of generalized neanderthaloids split into two divergent lines of evolution, one leading to the modern type of *Homo sapiens*, and the other to the extreme neanderthaloids that became extinct. But there are those who think that the neanderthaloids interbred with people of modern *Homo sapiens* type though, to my mind, this is no more than a speculative conjecture.

Still further back in time, during the second interglacial period, that is to say, about 200,000 years ago, *Homo sapiens* as represented by the generalized neanderthaloids was already in existence. This we know from parts of a skull found in 1935 and subsequent years twenty-four feet below the surface in well-stratified gravels at Swanscombe in the Thames Valley. Unfortunately only the bones forming the roof and back of the skull were found, but they were excellently preserved and my study of them revealed nothing unusual, as compared with modern skulls, with the main exception of their thickness. My collaborator, Dr G. M. Morant, who made a biometric comparison of the bones, also found nothing unusual about them. A subsequent statistical analysis, however, did show a minor differences from modern skulls in the dimensions of the occipital bone, but this difference is too slight to distinguish Swanscombe man from *Homo sapiens*. That the species *Homo sapiens* was already in existence 200,000 years ago was indeed an unexpected finding, but the age of the skull bones was very convincingly attested by the stratigraphical evidence, as well as by the evidence of the remains of extinct animals and the characteristic type of the stone implements found in association with them. Even so, the subsequent exposure of the Piltdown forgery raised doubts regarding its authenticity in the minds of some authorities, and it was here that the fluorine test proved so valuable. The test finally clinched the evidence, for the skull was found to contain just as great a concentration of fluorine as the bones of the extinct animals embedded in the same deposit.

Preceding *Homo sapiens* of the generalized neanderthaloid type there lived men of far more primitive appearance. The remains of these people were originally discovered in Java by a Dutch doctor, Eugene Dubois, in 1891, and the first discovered fossilized skull cap provoked the greatest interest and also a most vehement controversy. It showed such a remarkable combination of human and ape-like characters that Dubois gave to the type the name *Pithecanthropus*, which means 'ape-man'. The skull capacity was estimated to be not much more than 900 cubic centimetres—about twice that of the mean value of the modern large apes and only about two-thirds that of modern man. There was no rounded forehead, the eye-sockets were overhung by a shelf-like projecting brow ridge (as in some of the large apes) and, as subsequent discoveries showed, the nose was flattened and recessed, the jaws were massive and prominent with no chin and furnished with teeth of unusually large size. When the first discovery was announced some authorities suggested that the skull belonged to an extinct ape, a giant sort of gibbon; others maintained that it was definitely human; and yet others said it was neither, but a real 'missing link'. But the controversy, acrimonious as it was at the time, did not last very long. The size and shape of the brain (as determined by a cast of the inside of the skull—that is to say, an endocranial cast), and the discovery of a thigh bone quite similar to that of modern man, led to a common agreement that *Pithecanthropus* was definitely man and not ape. And this conclusion was later affirmed by a study of the dentition, for although the teeth were of large size, they conformed to the human pattern and not to the ape pattern. In addition, further remains of the same group were later found in China, a few miles from Pekin. These Chinese representatives of *Pithecanthropus* were more advanced than their Javanese cousins—they had somewhat larger brains (their cranial capacity was about 1,000 c.c. or more), the beginning of a rounded forehead, and an incipient chin eminence. They were also later in time, for while the Javanese fossils are reckoned, on the basis of potassium-argon dating, to have lived half a million years ago or so, the Chinese fossils probably date from about 400,000 years ago. In spite of their small brains and some of the 'simian' features of their skull and jaws, the Chinese pithecanthropines were evidently skilled hunters (the fossilized fragments of their prey have been found with their own remains), they were adept at making tools of rather a crude kind, and the remains of hearths make it clear that they knew how to make and use fire either to keep themselves warm or perhaps for culinary purposes. Whether the Javanese pithecanthropines fabricated stone implements we do not know for certain; it is likely that they did for crude implements have been found in deposits similar to those containing their skulls and jaws, but at a slightly higher stratigraphical level.

Evidently the pithecanthropines were not confined in their distribution to the Far East. Remains almost certainly attributable to the same type of primitive man have been found in Tanzania and in Algeria, both with an antiquity of something like half a million years. And in 1908 a massive, chinless jaw was found in a sandy deposit near Heidelberg, and its antiquity has also been estimated (on indirect geological evidence) to have been almost half a million years. We shall not know for certain until other parts of the skull and skeleton of 'Heidelberg man' have been discovered, but it seems likely enough that he was a European representative of the pithecanthropines. At any rate these ancient men were spread over a considerable area of the Old World in very early times. They showed a good deal of individual variation in their anatomical details, and there is an almost insensible gradation—forming a temporal as well as a structural sequence—leading from them through populations of the generalized neanderthal type to *Homo sapiens* of completely modern type. Incidentally, we may note that although the original pithecanthropine material was labelled by the scientific name *Pithecanthropus erectus* ('*erectus*' because the thigh bones made it clear that these people walked upright), the gradations leading to modern *Homo sapiens* are so closely continuous, and with so much overlapping in certain characters between the successive grades, that the term *'Pithecanthropus'* has been dropped, and we now use the scientific name *Homo erectus*. But, for the sake of convenience because of the long usage of the name with which they were first christened, we can still refer to the group by the colloquial name of the 'pithecanthropines'.

Without the need for dubious speculation, then, we may picture scattered populations of these remarkably primitive and small-brained pithecanthropines distributed over a large area of the Old World and already, half a million years ago, capable of making simple tools and weapons of stone. They may also have made wooden implements of some sort, but, if so, these would have rotted and disintegrated over such a vast period of time. The Chinese representatives of the group may also have made and used bone implements, for mixed up with their remains have been found sharp-pointed and sharp-edged splinters of animal bones. Some archaeologists have argued that these were artefacts deliberately shaped by human agency, but others have doubted whether this was so and take the view that the bone fragments are more likely to have been the broken remains of animal limb bones split open for their marrow content. The palaeolithic descendants of the pithecanthropines gradually improved their technique for fabricating stone implements by chipping and flaking, making hand-axes, choppers and so forth, but the development of this stone culture proceeded very slowly for many thousands of years and there was evidently a prolonged period of cultural stagnation until later palaeolithic man approaching the modern type of *Homo sapiens* began to make highly sophisticated flint tools such as sharp knives, scrapers, gravers and spear points or arrow heads, as well as articles of bone and antler. Towards the end of the Old Stone Age the delicate handiwork of these people produced articles of considerable beauty. No doubt the latter were the product of specialists who concentrated their time and skill on this kind of work. And the artistic activities of the cave-men of France were certainly the province of specialists also. Here we see the development of a division of labour in palaeolithic communities that in the course of time became a more pronounced feature of social organization, and still more so at the dawn of the neolithic period.

One of the curious features of the later stages of human evolution was the astonishing rapidity with which the brain became enlarged, for it increased in volume by about fifty per cent in half a million years. This rate of growth seems greatly to have exceeded that of anatomical characters generally in mammalian evolution. What was the reason for this? It can only be supposed that it was the resultant of extreme pressure of selection between competing communities, success in struggle for existence between them depending on enhanced intelligence and the latter demanding a more complex brain. This seems to be a natural inference, though surprisingly enough routine intelligence tests on *individuals* in modern communities have failed to show any marked correlation between brain size and intelligence. Perhaps this is due to the inadequacy of the intelligence tests, but we need to remember that in considering the evolution of the human brain we are dealing with mean values in *populations* and not with individual variations. It is probable that the pithecanthropine populations were distributed in comparatively small groups, living by hunting and foraging, and wandered from time to time in search of new territories. But, judging from the extensive concentrations of the products of their stone tool industries and their hunting activities, later palaeolithic communities must have been much larger. Moreover, with the successive glaciations of the Ice Age habitable regions and hunting territories would have become much more restricted, at any rate in what today are the temperate latitudes. It may be inferred, therefore, that, as the population density increased, there must have been quite a severe competition for living space between neighbouring or invading communities. Moreover, in order to contend with the vicissitudes of climate, palaeolithic man needed to exert all the faculties of his intelligence for the invention of tools and weapons to keep himself alive. Perhaps it was these times of strife and rivalry that stimulated the requirements for an increasing intelligence and greater inventive powers, and these, in turn, for the elaboration of a larger brain. This is an interesting conjecture, for it had long been supposed that it was primarily an increase in the size of the brain that determined the ability to develop cultures of greater complexity and greater efficiency, whereas the reverse may have been the case. Probably, however, it would be more correct to say that advancement in cultural organization and the enlargement of the brain proceeded pari passu with each other, the two interacting together in relation to the progressive demands of the environment.

We have noted that the pithecanthropines still preserved a number of simian characters in their skull, jaws and teeth, inherited, it is to be presumed, from their common ancestry with anthropoid apes. But whether, anatomically speaking, they should be regarded as representatives of the ape family rather than the family of mankind has depended not on their retention of simian characters but on the recognition that they had already, half a million years ago, developed features characteristic of the trend of evolution towards modern *Homo sapiens* and quite different from those characteristic of the trend of evolution that eventually led to the appearance of the modern apes. Taking into account these divergent trends of evolution what, we may hypothesize, would the still earlier precursors of the pithecanthropines have been like? It has long been accepted on the basis of many lines of evidence, that the ape family—Pongidae in zoological terms—and the family of mankind—

Hominidae—are the divergent products derived from a common ancestry. Indeed, their resemblances are so numerous that in zoological classification the two families are now grouped in a common 'super-family', the Hominoidea. But the modern pongids have been much more conservative in preserving archaic characters than the modern hominids, though the former also show divergent specializations that mark them off rather sharply from the latter. The divergence of the pongid and hominid trends of evolution from a common ancestral stock is generally accepted to have occurred a very long time ago, probably in the Miocene period of geology, that is to say at least 25 million years ago and perhaps even earlier. Now, the pithecanthropines lived sometime about the middle of the Pleistocene period, and it may be presumed, from what is known of the fossil records of other groups of mammals, that their evolutionary antecedents in the early part of the Pleistocene, one or two million years ago, would have been still more primitive and 'ape-like' in their anatomical characters. They would, one might have expected, have had still smaller brains and still larger jaws, but probably they would show features characteristic of the hominid trend of evolution in the details of their dentition as well as adaptations, no doubt still imperfect but nonetheless definite, for the upright posture and gait in which man so strongly contrasts with anthropoid apes. The remarkable thing is that this conjectural hypothesis has been verified by the discovery of just such primitive hominids in Africa. The first skull of these early types was found in limestone deposits in the Transvaal in 1924, and a preliminary note on it was published by Professor Raymond Dart of the Witwatersrand University in 1925. As with all discoveries of this kind, it led at first to considerable controversy, some of it rather unnecessarily contentious. Dart gave the name *Australopithecus* to the skull, a term meaning 'southern ape', but he pointed out that it showed a number of characters in which it made a much closer approach to hominids than to pongids. Very soon afterwards further remains of the same type were discovered by the late Dr Robert Broom in other parts of the Transvaal, confirming Dart's assessment of its hominid affinities. But the controversy still continued unabated.

In 1946 I visited South Africa to examine for myself all these fossils, and as further discoveries accumulated, I made further expeditions to examine them and to inspect the sites where they had been found. It was at this time that I became most reluctantly entangled in an unhappy dispute about the evolutionary significance of the *Australopithecus* group—or australopithecines as we may call them. Unhappy, because I deplore resorts to polemics in scientific discussions—polemics of any kind are quite inappropriate in discussions that should aim at an objective appraisal of evidence. But I was compelled to engage in this dispute, for the simple reason that some of my statements concerning the obvious hominid characters of the australopithecines were flatly contradicted on the basis of statistical comparisons. As it turned out, the statements made by my critics were not only based on inadequate statistical methods, they had also made a surprising arithmetical mistake in their statistical calculations. But they continued in their efforts to prove that the australopithecines did not differ materially in certain of their cranial and skeletal characters from the modern large apes though their statistical comparisons were in some cases vitiated by the fact that the measurements they made on the ape material and plaster casts of the australopithecine fossils were not always strictly comparable. Doubtless, such fallacies and misconstructions were nothing more than unfortunate oversights of essentials, but for a time they did confuse the issue on the real significance of these ancient hominids. Altogether, the history of these controversies makes a sad story, but it is surely an old story that may now be forgotten, for so many of the discoveries of the australopithecines in later years all went to confirm the conclusion that these were early representatives of the hominid line of evolution and quite distinct from the pongid line. Of course they were ape-like in the retention of primitive ancestral characters—'characters of common inheritance' as I have called them—just as their pithecanthropine successors still retained such characters though to a lesser degree. But these are not relevant to the question whether they should be classed in the family of the Pongidae rather than the family of the Hominidae. The relevant characters for deciding on this issue are those that were distinctive of the hominid trend of evolution in contrast to those that were distinctive of the pongid trend of evolution—what I have called 'characters of independent acquisition'. The mistake that my critics sometimes seem to have made in their attempts to assess the significance of the australopithecines was that they did not always distinguish between these two categories of anatomical characters. Or, to put the matter more succinctly, in technical terms they have been muddling up patristic with cladistic affinities. It was not so long ago that I read the astonishingly naive statement that it would be futile to attempt to argue whether or not a single morphological feature has, or has not, a greater evolutionary significance than another. But it is no doubt true to say that all those who are well experienced in the study of evolutionary trends by reference to fossil remains are agreed that incipient and progressive developments of morphological features which later become characteristic of a definitive group are of far greater importance for determining the evolutionary status of early types than any of the characters of common inheritance still retained from a common ancestry with allied groups. No, it is by no means futile—but it could be very fertile of error if morphological features were to be treated indiscriminately as though they were all of equal value in assessing the evolutionary status of extinct types of an intermediate kind; how simple then would be the task of determining evolutionary relationships—all could be accomplished with a pair of calipers and a digital computer! The fact is that statistical comparisons of different groups with the aim of establishing their mutual relationships are fraught with many difficulties, one of which involves the need to ensure that the anatomical characters compared are strictly equivalent with each other morphologically, and also that, so far as fossils are concerned, the measurements are made on original specimens and not on plaster casts of them. It also sometimes happens that measurements by one observer may not be made in quite the same way as those recorded by another. It was once remarked by Karl Pearson, a pioneer in the application of statistical methods to biological materials, that 'Science is measurement'. This aphorism states an obvious truth, but it is also true to say that not all measurements are scientific!

In spite of their small brains and large, powerful jaws, the australopithecines were furnished with a dentition of definitely human type, not only in the details of individual teeth but also in the pattern of their arrangement in the jaws and the flat kind of wear that they showed even in young individuals. Their milk teeth, also, were of human type. In spite of their small brains, again, the skull itself shows a number of characters that are typically hominid in contrast with ape skulls. For example, the vault of the cranium may be very high, the area for the attachment of the neck muscles on the back of the skull is quite restricted (whereas in the large anthropoid apes it is extensive to provide for the powerful neck muscles required for holding up the head which is held on a forwardly sloping spinal column), and the relatively forward position of the occipital condyles, that is, the joint surfaces on the base of the skull that articulate with the top of the spinal column, contrasts with their relatively backward displacement in the large apes. There are a number of other hominid features of the same sort, and it was some of these that first led to the supposition that in the australopithecines the head was more perfectly balanced on top of an approximately vertical spinal column than in apes (though not so nicely as it is in *Homo sapiens*), and that they had already achieved the upright stance and gait characteristic of hominids (though, again, not so efficiently as in modern man). These preliminary inferences regarding posture came to be strikingly confirmed by the subsequent discovery of australopithecine limb bones, including those of the pelvis. All these made it perfectly clear that the australopithecines were erect, bipedal creatures, but they also demonstrate that they had not attained to the proficiency of *Homo sapiens* in their ability to walk upright. The interesting thing is that these skeletal elements display just those intermediate characters that might be predicated for creatures already on the hominid line of evolution on its evolutionary travels, so to speak, from the presumed ancestral stock common to both ape and man. Of course, it is well known that the large apes, such as gorillas and chimpanzees, can erect themselves on their hind-limbs (as, indeed, some other mammals such as bears can do) and they can even walk a few steps. But this is not their usual mode of progression; on the ground they are normally quadrupedal, and in the trees they climb or swing among the branches with their elongated arms. The bones of their hind-limbs and their pelvis are very different from those of man, and they show none of the progressive and distinctively hominid traits of the australopithecines that betoken an advanced development towards the characteristically human posture and bipedal locomotion.

The australopithecine fossils to which I have been referring were mainly found in limestone caves and fissures in South Africa. It has not been possible to determine their exact antiquity, but archaeologists have expressed the opinion, on indirect evidence, that they date back to the early or middle part of the Pleistocene period, perhaps as much as half a million, or even a million, years ago. In 1959 Dr and Mrs Leakey discovered a practically complete australopithecine skull embedded deep down in well stratified deposits at the side of the impressive Olduvai gorge in Tanzania, and it proved possible to date this with considerable accuracy by the potassium-argon method; its age has been estimated by this method to be about one and three-quarter million years! It now begins to look as if the australopithecines appeared in East Africa a good deal earlier than those that occupied South Africa. We may hazard a guess, therefore, that some of them trekked down into the Transvaal and remained there as persistent relics perhaps long after more advanced hominids had already undergone an evolutionary development elsewhere.

What can we say of the status of the australopithecines? It might be misleading to refer to them as 'human' for we do not know whether they possessed attributes which in common parlance are associated with this term, such as the ability to talk and the inventive capacity for developing cultures of an elaborate kind. It is probably better to speak of them as representatives of the pre-human phase of hominid evolution. They were generally small in stature, they appear to have lived in hunting groups, for associated with their remains have been found layers of stalagmite packed tightly with the broken bones of animals on which they presumably fed, and, at least for much of the time they existed, they inhabited relatively arid country and not tropical forests such as are suitable for anthropoid apes. Even if they were not capable of symbolic speech, no doubt they possessed some degree of vocalization that would be needed for co-operative activities in their hunting pursuits. Perhaps, also, they were scavengers feeding on the remains of carcasses left by predatory carnivores. That they *used* tools such as stones and fragments of animal bones seems reasonably certain; even the modern apes do this sort of thing. But whether they actually *fabricated* tools and weapons has been the subject of much controversy. Some authorities have maintained that the animal bones found with their fossilized remains had been deliberately fashioned by them for use as implements, but not all agree with this interpretation. Crude stone artefacts, sometimes called pebble tools, have certainly been found in deposits closely associated with skeletal remains of the australopithecines, and even the flakes that had evidently been struck off in their manufacture. And we know that they had hands with well-developed opposable thumbs so that, anatomically speaking, they certainly had the manipulative capacity for fabricating stone or bone implements of a simple kind. I myself have taken the view, on the evidence so far available, that they did in fact make simple tools, but others are inclined to the view that the stone implements were perhaps made by more advanced types of hominid that lived contemporaneously with them, in spite of the fact that no indubitable remains of such advanced types with significantly larger brains have yet been found at the same sites. No doubt this debatable question will ultimately be solved by further excavations in South and East Africa.

The question now arises whether the small-brained australopithecines were ancestral to the pithecanthropines with their larger (but still rather small) brains. This seems likely enough, for the former certainly antedated the latter. Moreover, different groups of australopithecines showed considerable individual variability, and the jaws and teeth of some of the smaller, lightly-built individuals are not easily distinguishable from those of pithecanthropines that have been found in Java. But this is not to say that any of the australopithecines whose remains have so far been found were the actual *parents* of a line of descent that eventually gave rise to more advanced hominids; such an idea would be utterly absurd, for the chances of finding the fossil remains of actual ancestors, or even representatives of the local geographical group that provided the actual ancestors, are so remote as not to be worth consideration. But the fact is that in their anatomical structure the African fossils conform so closely to theoretical postulates for an intermediate phase of hominid evolution preceding the pithecanthropines as to lead to the inference that the australopithecine group as a whole, diversified as it was into different geographical varieties and perhaps even into different local species, somewhere or another provided the matrix, so to speak, from which more advanced hominids and eventually the species *Homo sapiens* itself derived their origin.

The australopithecines, as we have seen, were already in existence in the early part of the Pleistocene almost two million years ago. Were they preceded by even more ancient and still more primitive hominids? The evidence for this is still scanty and equivocal. We know that in Pliocene times, and the earlier Miocene period, there were many different kinds of anthropoid ape undergoing diversification in Africa and southern Asia. Among these was a fossil type known as *Ramapithecus* that extended its range from India to East Africa. Unfortunately it is known only from fragmentary jaws and parts of its dentition, but it has been suggested from the appearance of the teeth and their arrangement in the jaws that *Ramapithecus* was not an anthropoid ape strictly speaking, but a very early member of the hominid sequence of evolution after this line had diverged from the pongid sequence of evolution. If this interpretation should prove correct by the discovery of further and more complete remains, it would push that antiquity of man back ten or twenty million years, or even more. But while the fossil evidence allows us to speak with assurance on the antiquity of man as far back as the australopithecine phase in hominid evolution, further back than this we can at the moment only speculate rather hesitantly.

It was in 1863 that the famous geologist, Sir Charles Lyell, published the first edition of his remarkable classic *The Geological Evidence of the Antiquity of Man*. His evidence, based largely on the discoveries of remains of prehistoric man and his stone artefacts in river gravels that had evidently been deposited a very long time ago, and in geological formations that also contained the fossilized bones of extinct animals, was marshalled in such convincing detail that it became readily accepted by his fellow scientists and, indeed, excited the attention of many thoughtful laymen. That this was so is made clear by the fact that in the year of its publication the book ran into three editions, so great was the demand for it by the reading public. Lyell wrote that 'It is already clear that Man was contemporary in Europe with two species of elephant, now extinct, *E. primigenius* and *E. antiquus*, two also of rhinoceros, *R. tichorhinus* and *R. hemitoechus*, at least one species of hippopotamus, the cave-bear, cave-lion and cave-hyaena, various bovine, equine, and cervine animals now extinct, and many smaller Carnivora, Rodentia, and Insectivora.' Clearly he was thinking of the antiquity of man in terms of many thousands of years, but at that time he could hardly be more definite, and he goes on to say, 'We cannot ascertain at present the limits, whether of the beginning or the end, of the first stone period when Man co-existed with the extinct mammalia, but that it was of great duration we cannot doubt.' If he had been alive today, he would have expressed wonder at the evidence now available that the story of hominid evolution, a story recounted in a long and graduated series of fossil relics, can be traced back in terms not only of several thousand years but of a million years and more. But I doubt whether he would have been surprised, for it is evident from his book that he was contemplating the origin of the hominid line of evolution from an ape-like ancestor at a very remote time—perhaps as far back as the Pliocene or Miocene periods, and this, as we now know from our dating methods, would mean several million years ago.

CHAPTER 9

THE EXPOSURE OF THE PILTDOWN FORGERY

PILTDOWN Man, as he came to be known, was accepted as a genuine discovery of the highest importance by many authorities for many years. His supposedly great antiquity also led some to refer to him as the 'Earliest Englishman'. Reconstructions were modelled in the form of sculptured busts to show what he looked like in life, and these were put on view in a number of museums and figured in many authoritative textbooks dealing with human evolution. It is little wonder, then, that the exposure of the fraudulent nature of the fossil remains attributed to him led to wide excitement in the press. Looking back, it is a matter for surprise that some anthropologists at first expressed scepticism of the clearly overwhelming evidence that proved the whole discovery to be a fantastic piece of forgery, but this perhaps only serves to illustrate that even scientists of repute may sometimes find it difficult to abandon their preconceived ideas. As I mentioned in the previous chapter, it was the fluorine test that showed that the Piltdown fossils were not so very old after all. And it was my colleague Professor Weiner who demonstrated almost certainly the likelihood of a fraud by filing down and staining the teeth of a chimpanzee, thereby reproducing a remarkable resemblance to the apparently human type of flattening seen on the biting surface of the Piltdown molars.

In the investigation that followed I concentrated my attention on the purely anatomical evidence which seemed to me conclusive in itself to demonstrate that a forgery had been perpetrated. But I was only one of a team of specialists in many fields who applied one test after another corroborating the anatomical evidence. The combined results of all these studies amounted to the final proof of an incredible imposture. In 1955, I was invited to deliver a lecture at the Royal Institution on these results, and in this chapter, with the kind permission of the Director of the Institution, I am reproducing this lecture which, for me, was a notable occasion. The story of the exposure of this amazing archaeological hoax is now an old story, but I think it is a story well worth the re-telling.

*   *   *   *   *   *

The discovery of parts of a human skull and an ape-like jaw in a gravel deposit at Piltdown in Sussex some forty years ago led many authorities to the conclusion that they were the remains of a very archaic and lowly type of man—possibly an ancestral type which gave rise during the course of later evolution to modern *Homo sapiens*. It was given the name *Eoanthropus*, or the Dawn Man. As we now know, the whole discovery was entirely based on a most elaborate fabrication of the evidence, and it is probably true to say that the Piltdown forgery was the greatest archaeological hoax of its kind ever perpetrated. To those who read the account of the exposure of this forgery, three questions must have come to mind at once— (1) How came it that so many distinguished scientists were deluded for so many years? (2) What first led to the discovery of the forgery? (3) Who was the actual forger? With the last question I shall not deal. But it is a question which has made quite necessary a good deal of detailed enquiry, not so much because it is important to know who was the culprit, but because it obviously is a matter of importance—in order completely to exonerate others of all trace of suspicion—to know who could *not* have been the culprits. The fact is that a number of eminent scientists who took part in the excavations at Piltdown and in the original study of the remains have been shown by this enquiry to have been entirely innocent (as, indeed, might have been anticipated from their long record of personal and scientific integrity).

How came it, then, that so many distinguished scientists were misled for so long? Let me briefly recount the main facts of the first discovery. Early in 1912 some fragments of a human skull were brought by Mr Charles Dawson to Dr (later Sir Arthur) Smith Woodward of the Department of Geology in the Natural History Museum. Charles Dawson was a solicitor practising in Lewes, who in his spare time was an enthusiastic antiquarian. He had conducted a number of excavations on neolithic sites, Roman earthworks and so forth, and he had had a long experience of collecting fossils over the Sussex Weald. According to Dawson, the skull fragments had in the first instance been found by workmen who were carting gravel from Piltdown. The bones were unusually thick and appeared to be well mineralized. Smith Woodward joined in systematic excavations at the site and later, with the help of Dawson, found further portions of the brain-case and half of a lower jaw. These specimens were all found close together—within a few feet of each other—and the jaw and a part of the occipital bone were reported to have been discovered *in situ* (that is, it was assumed, in undisturbed gravel). All the pieces were conspicuously iron-stained, as was to be expected in fossil bones which had become naturally embedded in the ferruginous Piltdown gravels.

Smith Woodward pieced together the bones of the brain-case and was thus able to reconstruct the skull as it presumably appeared when it was complete, and he fitted to it the ape-like lower jaw. From the first there were a few critics who found it difficult to suppose that so ape-like a jaw could belong to the skull, for the jaw socket in the temporal bone of the skull was of typically human conformation and might be assumed, therefore, to have articulated with a jaw of essentially human type. In fact, however, there were at the time very strong arguments for the conclusion that both the brain-case and the jaw belonged to the same individual.

Smith Woodward's original reconstruction of the brain-case showed it to possess a number of features which were very primitive, and even simian, in character. For example, it was low-vaulted and the cranial capacity was unusually small. Moreover, Elliot Smith (who was then Professor of Anatomy at University College, London, and accepted as an outstanding authority on the anatomy and evolution of the human brain) studied an endocranial cast of Smith Woodward's reconstructed skull, and on the basis of this he made the pronouncement that the brain of 'Piltdown man' was the most primitive and simian human brain ever recorded. On the other hand, although the lower jaw was obviously simian in shape (particularly in the chin region) with molars of simian proportions, the teeth had been worn down flat on their biting surfaces in human fashion and, from their X-ray appearance, were said to show quite short roots (in contrast to the much longer roots which are typical of apes' molars). The wear of the teeth appeared to demonstrate quite clearly that the movements of the jaw in mastication must have been similar to those of man, and very different from anthropoid apes in which the projecting and interlocking canine teeth limit free rotatory and side-to-side movements. A cranium of general human appearance but with some ape-like features, and a jaw and teeth of general ape-like appearance but with some human features, clearly seemed to harmonize with each other.

It should be noted that, when the lower jaw was first described by Smith Woodward, he postulated that the canine tooth belonging to it must have been of a simian type in its general proportions, but that it could not have projected and interlocked with the canine of the upper jaw (otherwise the molar teeth could not have become worn so flat), and that it must have shown a rather unusual type of wear. He made a reconstruction of the canine as, according to his reasoning, it must have appeared. The extraordinary thing is that, a few months later, a canine tooth was found in the excavations at Piltdown which proved to be, in its shape and the nature of its wear, almost exactly like the reconstructed tooth. At the time, of course, the discovery was regarded as a remarkable vindication of the methods and the lines of reasoning of the anatomists who had postulated a canine tooth of such construction. We now know that it has a more sinister interpretation.

As I have already mentioned, some authorities did doubt the natural association of the Piltdown brain-case with the Piltdown jaw, and assumed that, as the result of a most astonishing coincidence, a fossil human skull of primitive type had happened to become juxtaposed side by side with the jaw of a hitherto unknown type of extinct ape. But even this interpretation was regarded by many as entirely excluded by a second discovery reported to Smith Woodward by Dawson in 1915. This discovery, said to have been made in a field about two miles from the first Piltdown site, consisted of a small piece of a frontal bone (quite similar in thickness and texture to the original skull), a fragment of an occipital bone, and an isolated molar tooth identical in shape and proportions with the molar teeth of the jaw (but not so severely worn). That a *second* coincidence of the association of fragments of a human brain-case with a tooth of ape-like proportions could occur seemed out of the question, and many of those who were critical of Smith Woodward's interpretation of the Piltdown skull and jaw were converted to his point of view.

Thus all the anatomical evidence appeared to be quite consistent. It also appeared to be consistent with the geological evidence. The gravel deposit at Piltdown is situated in the valley of the Ouse, at some height above the level of the present river. It was stated to correspond to the 100-foot river terrace system (a statement which was accepted by such eminent geologists as Sollas and Boyd Dawkins), and since the 100-foot terrace system was formed in the earlier part of the Pleistocene period, this implied a considerable antiquity for the Piltdown skull and jaw. Such a conclusion apparently received full corroboration from the remains of extinct mammals also found in the Piltdown gravels, e.g. teeth of the Early Pleistocene *Elephas planifrons*, and of *Rhinoceros* and *Mastodon*. Some extremely crude flint implements from the same site were taken to indicate, also, a very primitive stage of palaeolithic culture. Lastly, it must be mentioned that scrapings of one of the cranial bones were removed for the analysis of organic matter, and the latter was found to be practically absent; in other words, the bone was evidently well fossilized.

From this brief account, it will be seen that all the collateral lines of evidence appeared to be mutually confirmatory and in complete harmony with each other—so much so, indeed, that (as we now realize) none of the experts concerned were led to examine their own evidence as critically as otherwise they certainly would have done. If any inconsistencies had appeared at this stage of the investigation, it can hardly be doubted that suspicions might have been raised. For example, if a detailed geological survey had then been available to show (as it did some years later) that the Piltdown gravel is really part of the 50-foot terrace and thus no more ancient than the latter part of the Pleistocene, the evidence of the fossil elephant and the mastodon would certainly have been scrutinized more carefully. Or if the canine tooth had shown the type of wear characteristic of modern apes (thus indicating an interlocking of the canines of upper and lower jaws), the nature of the wear of the molar teeth would have been more critically questioned. Or if the organic content of the Piltdown jaw had been analysed and found to be (as we now know is the case) as high as in a modern ape's jaw, the detection of the forgery would have been almost certain. You may think that the failure to estimate the organic matter in the jaw was rather a serious omission. But the jaw and some of the cranial bones had been found in the gravel deposit by experienced workers in immediate proximity to each other and showed the same degree of iron-staining, and there was thus no reason to suppose at that time that they had different origins. The cranial bone used for the nitrogen analysis was taken as a sample of the whole collection of specimens, and in any case there would have been a natural reluctance to mutilate what was presumed to be a quite unique specimen by drilling holes in the jaw in order to get material for analysis.

As a matter of fact, a rather serious discrepancy in the otherwise harmonious evidence did appear soon after the publication of the original report on the Piltdown discovery. Professor (later Sir Arthur) Keith, Conservator of the Museum of the Royal College of Surgeons, detected a remarkable mistake in Smith Woodward's reconstruction of the brain-case. It was a mistake which was no doubt excusable for anyone not thoroughly well versed in the finer details of human osteology (Smith Woodward himself, of course, was not a human anatomist), but it had rather far-reaching effects. He had mistaken a small side ridge on the roof of the skull for a *median* ridge(such as is not uncommon in ancient human skulls), and as a result his reconstruction of the Piltdown skull made it appear unusually primitive in its general form and with an unusually small brain. Keith's correction of this error showed quite clearly that the brain-case was in fact entirely similar in proportions to a modern human cranium and that the cranial capacity was well within the range of that of modern man. Why, it may be asked, did not this correction immediately raise suspicions of the authenticity of the Piltdown fossils? I regret to record that it most unfortunately gave rise to a rather acrimonious, and somewhat painful, controversy between Keith and Elliot

Smith, and because of its personal nature the controversy certainly clouded the issues and befogged the atmosphere of scientific discussion. Elliot Smith failed to recognize the true significance of Keith's correction, and, in spite of it, still maintained that the skull and brain did show markedly primitive and simian characters, while the ape-like characters of the jaw, in his view, had been exaggerated. In his day Elliot Smith's authority carried great weight (and rightly so, for he was a very eminent anatomist), so that not only did he persuade himself that his original interpretation of the skull and endocranial cast had been fundamentally right, he also seems to have persuaded biologists in general that this was so. I cannot help supposing that if Smith Woodward had not made the initial error in the reconstruction of the skull, or if the error had been freely recognized by all those concerned as soon as it was pointed out by Keith, the evidence of the skull and jaw might have been seriously reconsidered and all the collateral evidence reassessed, with the possibility that the forgery might have been exposed at that time.

But the controversy following Keith's disclosure did lead to a crystallization of two main schools of opinion: (1) those who continued to maintain that the skull and jaw belonged to the same creature, *Eoanthropus*, and (2) those who still held that the skull was that of a fossil type of man, and the jaw that of an early and hitherto unknown type of extinct ape. There were others, also, who preferred to put on one side the whole series of specimens as inadequate for drawing any firm conclusions, pending the discovery of further and more complete material. No-one at that time, including those who most strongly criticized the original interpretations put forward by Smith Woodward and Elliot Smith, ever suggested the possibility of a forgery. Even Keith himself accepted the conclusion that the skull and jaw belonged to the same individual, though he never ceased to express himself as puzzled about this curious combination of a modern-sized brain with a simian type of jaw.

There is one point which I should like to stress here. It has been recently suggested that the Piltdown forgery might have been detected by some of the experts of the time if they had had more opportunity of studying the original specimens (rather than casts), the implication being that Smith Woodward was too secretive about the specimens and was reluctant to allow them to be inspected by his colleagues. That this is quite untrue is shown by a letter which Keith published in *Nature* in 1913 in which he said, 'Anatomists have had no difficulty in gaining the freest access to the actual specimens; even those who, like myself, regard the original reconstruction of the skull and brain-cast as fundamentally erroneous, have had every privilege granted to them on repeated visits to see the Piltdown fragments in Dr Smith Woodward's keeping.'

We now come to the next phase in the puzzle of the Piltdown discovery, about five years ago [i.e. 1950], when Dr Kenneth Oakley of the British Museum had been developing and applying the fluorine test for estimating the relative antiquity of fossils. This test depends on the fact that, when a fossil bone or tooth becomes embedded in a porous deposit (such as gravel), in the course of time it takes up fluorine ions from the minute traces of this element which may be present in the percolating water and part of its substance becomes converted into a very stable compound, fluorapatite. The longer the fossil remains embedded in the deposit, the greater the amount of fluorine will it contain. Thus the amount of fluorine present in a fossil bone or tooth may give an approximate indication of its relative antiquity. Oakley applied his test to the Piltdown specimens and, to his surprise, found that the fluorine content was so small in the skull, jaw and teeth, that it was clear they could not be older than the latter part of the Pleistocene period, and were perhaps even younger than that. This revelation called attention to a geological survey map of the Piltdown area which had been prepared some years earlier by Dr F. H. Edmunds of the Geological Survey, from which it became certain that the Piltdown gravels belong, not to the 100-foot terrace system as originally stated, but to the much younger 50-foot terrace system which dates from the latter part of the Pleistocene. This at once posed some most awkward questions. Either it had to be supposed that a most peculiar type of man with an ape-like jaw was living in Europe contemporaneously with the completely modern type of man represented by the later Palaeolithic communities, or it had to be supposed that the cranial bones were those of a modern type of man, while the jaw bone was that of an unknown type of extinct ape which somehow had managed to penetrate into northern Europe in spite of the severe climatic vicissitudes of the Ice Age. Either of these alternatives seemed to make nonsense. Then in 1953, my colleague, Dr Weiner, following some discussions on the whole perplexing conundrum of Piltdown, put forward the proposition that the only possible interpretation which could explain all the paradoxes and inherent contradictions of the Piltdown skull and jaw was that the jaw really belonged to a modern ape and had been deliberately faked and stained to simulate fossil specimens and subsequently 'planted' near the skull bones in the Piltdown gravel. But there appeared to be one main objection to this startling suggestion—the flat wear of the molar teeth at such an early stage of attrition (a type of wear not found in any of the modern apes). Dr Weiner then took a chimpanzee jaw, filed down the molar teeth to form flat biting surfaces and stained them with potassium permanganate. When he showed the results of his experiment to me the next morning I looked at the teeth with amazement, for they reproduced so exactly the appearance of the unusual type of wear in the Piltdown molars. We therefore took the first opportunity to visit the Natural History Museum in London in order to examine the original Piltdown specimens with the possibility in mind that the teeth had been flattened by artificial abrasion. But we first had to consider what were the features by which the effects of natural wear of a tooth might be expected to differ from the effects of artificial abrasion. A study of a large series of human and ape teeth showed us that there were a certain number of features on which we could probably place reliance, and when we inspected the Piltdown molars in the light of this experience the evidences of artificial abrasion immediately sprang to the eye. Indeed, so obvious did they seem that it may well be asked—how was it that they had escaped notice before? The answer is really quite simple—they had never been looked for. The history of scientific discovery is replete with examples of the obvious being missed because it had not been looked for, and the present instance is just one more example; nobody previously had ever examined the Piltdown jaw with the idea of a possible forgery in mind.

If the partially worn lower molar teeth in human or ape jaws are examined, certain rather consistent characteristics will be noted: (1) The first molar tooth is normally more severely worn than the second, for the reason that it erupts much earlier and is thus exposed to several years of wear before the second comes into use. (2) The molar teeth of the lower jaw wear down more severely on the outer than the inner side, for the reason that in normal occlusion of the teeth the upper molars overlap the outer margins of the lower molars. (3) When the enamel has been worn off the summits of the cusps, the underlying dentine is exposed and, being less hard in consistency, it becomes worn more rapidly by normal attrition. At this stage of wear, therefore, the exposed areas of dentine form shallow concavities, depressed below the level of the surrounding enamel. (4) The worn biting surfaces of adjacent molar teeth normally form part of a uniform contour since they function as a unit in chewing movements backward and forward and side-to-side. (5) The margins of the worn surfaces are usually rounded and bevelled as the result of the grinding movements against the cusps of the upper molar teeth.

An examination of the Piltdown molars immediately brought to view some very significant features: (1) The first and second molars are worn to almost exactly the same degree. (2) Much more dentine is exposed on the inner than on the outer cusps; in other words, the greater wear is on the inner side of the molars —*the wrong way round*. (3) The exposed areas of dentine are quite flat with the surrounding enamel (instead of forming shallow concavities). (4) The worn surfaces appear to be *too* flat for normal wear, and their margins are sharp and unbevelled (5) The surfaces of the two molars are out of alignment with each other and do not combine to form a harmonious contour, and that this is not the result of a post-mortem displacement of the teeth is seen in an X-ray photograph which clearly shows the 'contact facets' of the two molars in their proper apposition. (6) New X-ray photographs show that, contrary to the earlier reports, the roots of the molars are quite similar to those of apes in their length and disposition. (7) Close inspection of the biting surfaces of the molars with a binocular microscope reveals that they are scored with criss-cross scratches, apparently the result of the application of an abrasive of some sort. All these items of evidence, added together, led to the certain conclusion that the flat wear of the molar teeth was not the result of natural attrition but of a deliberate fabrication.

Now let us turn to the canine tooth. I have already mentioned that the nature of the wear on this tooth is unusual; it is, in fact, quite unlike that seen in either man or apes. It is confined to the inner surface of the crown, and over the whole of this surface from the anterior to the posterior border of the tooth the entire thickness of the enamel has been worn away, exposing the underlying dentine. But this advanced degree of wear is hardly compatible with the evident fact that the tooth is a young tooth which had either not yet completed its eruption or had only quite recently done so. This fact is established by X-ray photographs which show that the pulp cavity is relatively large, and apparently still widely open at the apex of the root. In the centre of the exposed dentine is a small patch of somewhat different appearance; this was stated in 1913 by the late Professor Underwood (a dental authority) to be secondary dentine. Now this statement assumes some importance when one remembers that secondary dentine is formed in a tooth as a reaction to natural attrition, and it would therefore mean that the wear on the Piltdown canine was indeed the result of natural attrition. But we now know that the patch in the middle of the exposed dentine is not secondary dentine at all —it marks a place where an opening has been made (presumably inadvertently) into the pulp cavity and has been plugged with a plastic material of some sort. The X-ray photograph, in fact, shows no evidence of the deposition of any secondary dentine which might have been expected to have resulted from the severe wear of the canine if this had been the result of natural attrition during life. There are several other points of interest in the canine tooth. For example, its abraded surface (like the flat surfaces of the molars) shows an abundance of fine scratches which suggests the application of an abrasive agent. Again, the X-ray photograph shows that the pulp cavity is filled with grains of sand, giving an appearance which strongly forces on one an impression of a prolonged period of fossilization during which the tooth, being rolled about in the river bed of the Ouse, gradually became infiltrated through the apex of its pulp cavity with sandy material. But a closer study has demonstrated (1) that the sand grains are loose and have not become cemented together in a ferruginous matrix (which would be expected if fossilization had occurred in the Piltdown gravels), and (2) the sand grains are of *the wrong size*. The fact is that, although these grains have been shown to be similar in composition to the sandy component of the Piltdown gravels, they are practically all about 1-2 mm. in diameter, whereas the sand at Piltdown contains an abundance of much finer material. If, therefore, the sand grains had been washed into the pulp cavity of the canine by natural agencies, they would be expected to be mixed with this finer silt. Perhaps the most remarkable thing about the Piltdown canine is its dark-brown and black discoloration. This had been assumed to be due to an iron incrustation over the surface—the result of being for so long embedded in the ferruginous Piltdown gravels. But this surface film did not throw a shadow on the X-ray photographs, and it has been analysed at the Research Laboratory of the National Gallery and found to be a bituminous paint—almost certainly Vandyke brown!

The anatomical evidence of the molar teeth and the canine found at Piltdown was, in my opinion, sufficient to demonstrate that their peculiar type of wear had been deliberately faked. Indeed, it was this evidence which led us to further enquiries by subjecting the jaw and teeth to a detailed chemical and physical examination by a number of different techniques. For the purpose of estimating the content of nitrogen (which provides an index of the amount of organic matter present) and of fluorine and certain other elements, material was obtained by drilling into the skull bones and the jaw and teeth. When the technical expert of the Natural History Museum drilled into the jaw, he was astonished to perceive a smell as of 'burning horn'. Clearly the bone had not undergone complete fossilization—it was, it seems, still comparatively recent! In contrast, the drilling of the skull bones was accompanied by no smell of burning. The skull bones, again, only produced a fine powder when drilled, whereas the jaw produced 'shavings' just like a fresh bone. The production of bone shavings rather than bone powder depends on the persistence of the organic fibrous matrix, which preserves the essential texture of the fresh bone. This fibrous tissue was identified later by examination with the electron microscope, though in the skull bones no trace of the tissue could be found by this method. It is not possible on this occasion to go into all the details of the chemical and physical analysis of the bones, but a very brief reference may be made to some of the findings. The organic matter in the Piltdown jaw and teeth was found to be as high as it is in the jaws and teeth of modern apes, and the fluorine content negligible. Further investigation by means of X-ray spectrophotometry and chemical tests demonstrated that the jaw had been stained with a bichromate solution, evidently in an attempt to match the natural staining which would be expected to follow a long period of deposition in the Piltdown gravel. All this sort of evidence, of course, entirely confirmed the anatomical evidence that the Piltdown jaw and teeth are deliberate fakes.

In the early stage of our investigations we had supposed that only the jaw and teeth might be fraudulent. But the exposure of this forgery directed attention to the other remains stated to have been found at Piltdown, and these later enquiries led to the startling conclusion that every one of them had been 'planted' in order to provide a complex framework of complementary evidence for the supposed antiquity of the skull and jaw. The skull bones themselves, although partly fossilized (but probably not very ancient), were found by X-ray crystallography to contain a quantity of gypsum, or calcium sulphate, which had been formed in the course of artificial staining with an iron sulphate solution (again, to match the colour of the Piltdown gravels). The remains of the extinct animals reported to have come from Piltdown had obviously been derived from other sources (as particularly clearly demonstrated by radiometric analysis and the fluormetric estimation of uranium). The so-called flint implements had likewise been stained with iron and bichromate solutions to match the local flint, and the stain was found by the application of hydrochloric acid to be entirely superficial. The unique bone implement found at

Piltdown, fashioned from the thigh bone of a fossil elephant, was shown by experimental tests to have been quite certainly shaped with a steel knife—for the cut surfaces at its end could not possibly have been produced by a flint implement (as had been supposed). Finally, the Piltdown gravels are now known to have a degree of acidity which makes it very difficult to suppose that any fossil bones could remain in them for any considerable period of time without undergoing decalcification.

I have told you something of the story of the detection of the Piltdown forgery. It is a story which has a number of different aspects, depending on the way in which you look at it. It has a tragic aspect when you consider it in the light of human frailty and the intentions behind the deliberate deception, and when you consider the unhappy controversies and personal estrangements to which the 'discoveries' gave rise. It gives one a furious sense of anger when one thinks of the hours and weeks and months of wasted time spent on the study of these bogus fossils. It has (let us admit it) a distinctly humorous aspect, for there is undoubtedly something that titillates our sense of the ridiculous in the idea of learned men being, so to speak, 'led up the garden path' by the skill and cunning of a hoaxer. It has a melancholy aspect when one remembers that the late Sir Arthur Smith Woodward, on his retirement, went to live near Piltdown in order to continue excavations there, which he did for a number of years until failing health prevented him from continuing his search. Of course, he did not find anything, for the fact is (and you may put what construction you like on it, though your construction on this fact alone will not necessarily be the right one) that after Charles Dawson's illness and death in 1916, that is to say, after Dawson ceased to play any part in the excavations at Piltdown, no fossils have ever been found in the gravel deposits there—the latter are apparently quite unfossiliferous. But the story of Piltdown also has a positive

CPE Q

aspect. For the detection of the forgery has led to the development and perfection of a whole battery of techniques which will in future be of the greatest use in estimating the antiquity of genuine fossils. They will also make it virtually impossible for anyone ever to repeat a similar deception again. Indeed, I venture to say that if Dr Oakley, Dr Weiner and myself, knowing all we know now about methods of forging fossil specimens, and with the assistance of all those scientists who have helped in the analysis of the Piltdown specimens, made full use of our knowledge, even we would not be skilful enough to perpetrate a forgery which would be incapable of detection by these refined techniques.

I said at the beginning of my discourse that the Piltdown forgery was the greatest archaeological hoax of its kind ever perpetrated. When I made this comment to a rather cynical friend of mine, he replied, 'What you really mean, of course, is that the Piltdown forgery is the greatest archaeological hoax of its kind which has so far been found out!' Well, some of the techniques have already been applied to some human remains which have been generally accepted on geological evidence to be of a high antiquity, and these remains have passed their tests quite satisfactorily.

CHAPTER 10

ISLANDS AND MOUNTAINS AND RIVERS

WHEN a small child is taken to the seaside he commonly finds one of his greatest enjoyments in piling up a mountain of sand with a surrounding moat, and then constructing a valley to let the incoming tide flow up like a river and convert the mountain into an island. Standing on the top of his mountain he delights in all the thrills of watching the approach of a flowing river, and all the sense of detachment that goes with isolation and the feeling of domination that goes with height. These attitudes of mind are complementary to each other, and the conjunction of islands and mountain tops and rivers in a common theme is thus not so incongruous as at first sight they might seem to be.

Whenever I land on a small island I feel I am stepping on a mountain top, for many oceanic islands are the tops of mountains whose base has in the course of ages become submerged far below the sea. A chain of islands likewise marks the denticulate peaks of a mountain range once elevated majestically to the skies from a surface of dry land, but now for the most part concealed beneath the water. The submergence of a mountain allows one to reach its summit lazily by boat instead of struggling up its slopes for a matter of perhaps several thousand feet, but in their geological genesis the island and the mountain partake of essentially the same nature.

Whenever I reach the top of a mountain I feel I am on an island, and, looking down on rolling undulations of the ground far below, I can almost imagine them as the heaving of the sea stilled in a momentary pause. Biologically speaking, I am indeed on an island, for, as everyone knows, above

227

certain altitudes the climatic environment can no longer accommodate the types of animals and plants and trees that are adapted to lowland districts—it carries its own characteristic fauna and flora isolated from those of neighbouring peaks by the intervening country.

Both mountains and islands have played a similar role in promoting the evolution of diverse types of animals and plants by separating one group of an ancestral population from another; thus such groups can no longer interbreed and no longer by freely intermingling their common genetic characters sustain the homogeneity of the common type. The importance of this factor of geographical isolation for evolutionary diversification is of course well recognized. Many years ago Charles Darwin, during the voyage of the *Beagle*, noted that in the different islands of the Galapagos archipelago off the west coast of Ecuador the finches are distinguished by differences in plumage and other characters; they had evidently undergone divergent trends of evolutionary development following their prolonged isolation from each other. In fact, it was this particular example of geographical variation that provided one of the most cogent arguments in Darwin's thesis of the origin of species. In our own country we have the British red deer and the St. Kilda's wren, that have been distinguished by some zoologists from their continental relations as distinct species or subspecies even though, as we know from geological data, the British Isles have only been separated from the Continent by water for about eight or nine thousand years. In Malaysia the little mouse deers that inhabit the large territories of Borneo or Sumatra are all of the same type, but in the compact group of islands between Singapore and the southern part of Sumatra— islands that can hardly have been isolated from the mainland for a very long time—no less than seven different varieties or subspecies of this small mammal have been distinguished. The island of Madagascar, long cut off from the mainland of

Africa, is perhaps one of the most outstanding demonstrations
of the effects of insular isolation on the emergence of novel
forms of life; many of the animals living there, or which used
to live there but are now extinct, have developed types of a
curious and aberrant nature such as are not to be found anywhere else in the world.

The flora and fauna of individual mountains, left standing as
'islands' on dry land, may show a similar diversification of
living creatures consequent on their isolation at high altitudes.
For example, the genus *Capra*, better known as the ibex, is to
be found on mountains of the Alps, the Caucasus, Abyssinia,
and elsewhere, but in each territory they have in course of time
become so different from each other that they have come to be
regarded as distinct species. Even more striking, I think, is the
fact that butterflies occupying mountain heights that have in
the geological past become separated from each other by the
erosion of deep valleys in what was once a common table-land
have in some cases been diversified into different varieties or
subspecies; they have become so intimately adapted to the
environmental conditions of their own particular mountain,
and the hazards of flight from one peak to another are so severe,
that the chances of interbreeding are practically eliminated.

But let me return to a few of my island memories. In my
boyhood days some of the best adventure stories were centred
on desert islands—we read Defoe's *Robinson Crusoe*, Marryat's
Masterman Ready, Ballantyne's *The Coral Island*, Stevenson's
Treasure Island, and suchlike books. I do not suppose that boys
of the present generation still find these stories as enthralling as
we did; probably not—the imaginative ideas engendered by
this era of space travel have led to a spate of boys' books
embodying so-called science fiction, but to my mind these are
too unrealistic to make satisfying reading. Perhaps the youth
of today would not altogether agree with me. They may well
argue that adventure stories of wrecks on desert islands have

themselves now become unrealistic, partly because there are fewer desert islands available for occupation by marooned voyagers, and partly because with modern means of communication no ship is likely to be wrecked off a coast without the rapid detection of its whereabouts. I once had occasion myself to explore a desert island, or, I should better say, an uninhabited island, for it displayed all the luxuriance of tropical vegetation. It was a small island a few miles off the coast of Borneo. It had a white sandy beach banked up behind with rows of tall coconut palms, and rising up beyond these was a wooded hill reaching a height of almost 700 feet. Attractive in all aspects, it really was a miniature of the 'desert island' of my boyhood fiction. As I surveyed it from its central hill, it seemed to me a most delightful island on which to be wrecked as a castaway if one ever had to endure such a fate. There was a light intermittent breeze that gently swayed the fronds of the coconut palms in synchronous flutters, and the waves streaked lazily into little breakers on a small fringing reef of coral near the shore. I fell to contemplating whether it could by itself support one or two ship-wrecked mariners for any length of time. There was plenty of wood to construct a shelter or for making fires, there was a fresh water supply from a spring on the side of the hill, there were coconuts and wild figs and occasional turtles' eggs to eat, and maybe some turtles to be caught. But I decided that in order to survive it would be necessary to depend largely on a fish diet. This would not be too difficult to obtain for I had had some experience with native methods of fishing. For example there were the jala-jala nets of the Malays—cast-nets circular in shape and several yards in diameter, with a series of stones or bits of iron as weights round the circumference. I had found that it requires a good deal of practice to throw a net of this sort; it is held bunched up near the centre and swung round, and it has to be cast in such a way that the weights all touch the water simultaneously. As they sink the edges of the net are drawn together by the weights and thus trap any fish that may have been covered by the casting. Then there was the small seine net, or pukat, that needs to be manipulated by two people wading into the sea, one of them circling as far out as practicable and then the two dragging the net by each end up to the shore. These essays of mine with the pukat had often brought successful catches. And I knew how to make a fire by the Dyak method of twirling a pointed stick of wood rapidly on a fixed log with a little hollow filled with wood shavings. Yes, I thought, I should be able to manage quite well. Particularly if I had a very companionable companion with me on my island.

Flying over islands at a height of one or two thousand feet emphasizes the reality that they are commonly isolated tops of mountains left exposed by the submergence of their foundations, for one can often see in the clear waters of tropical seas the sloping flanks of the mountains fading away translucently into the depths. I have seen this appearance among the little islands of the South China Sea, and once also on a flight along the island chain stretching from Java to Timor. But the most vivid expression of this phenomenon is to be seen when flying over the Great Barrier Reef of Australia. The view from the air of coral islands and atolls is exquisitely beautiful. The vivid green of the vegetation on the islands is surrounded by the sparkling whiteness of a coral beach, and then by a halo of delicate greens and blues looking like the iridescent colours of the ocellus of a peacock's feather glistening in the sunlight, but even more luminous and more subtle in their gradations. This encircling nimbus of successive blendings of colour is, of course, the result of the progressive deepening of the water around the submerged slopes of the height that remains above the sea-level to form the coral island. I have read some of the argumentative discussions by various authorities on the origins of coral islands in general, and of the Great Barrier Reef in particular. The explanation propounded by Darwin during the voyage of the *Beagle* seems now to have been for the most part confirmed by deep borings—that in the first instance a fringing reef of coral develops around the shores of an island, and that a gradual subsidence of the island is accompanied by the continuous upgrowth of corals keeping pace with the submergence and leading to the formation of the encircling barrier reef. The fact is that the polyps that form the calcareous matrix of coral are not able to live beyond a depth of about thirty fathoms and, following the gradual submergence to greater depths, the coral-forming animalcules that perish leave behind them, as a legacy to their successors, a compact mass of the calcareous formations they have constructed on top of which a new generation of polyps can continue to build living coral.

A visit for even a few days to a coral island will always remain vividly in the memory. I was able to enjoy such an experience in 1952 when I was in Queensland on a tour of Australian universities. I stayed on a small island, small enough to allow me to explore it thoroughly during my short stay. It was closely packed in the centre with trees—tall pisonias with light grey trunks and a tender green foliage, here and there groups of pandanus trees, or 'screwpines', perched up on divided roots splayed out like stilts and with their characteristic fruit of superficially pineapple appearance, a fringe of scattered casuarinas, and clumps of stately coconut palms. The surrounding beach was startlingly white in the sunlight. At one end of the island was the wreck of an old ship calling attention to the fact that coral islands and coral reefs have a sinister as well as an exquisitely beautiful aspect. Between the outer barrier reef and the beach at low tide was a lagoon—not strictly speaking a lagoon I have been told, for this term is more properly applied to the central water enclosed by a coral atoll that remains exposed at high tide, whereas our own outer barrier reef then became submerged. But even at high tide the extent of the submerged coral reef within the barrier was clearly to be seen because of the bright turquoise blue of its water contrasting with the deep ultramarine of the sea beyond. At any rate I took it as a lagoon, for so it appeared to me at low tide, and it was then that I could wade about in it and explore for myself its multicoloured garden of living coral. Coral fish of fantastic shapes and colours parade amidst this garden, bêches-de-mer of various sizes and patterns, nudibranchs with the most delicate tints that swim in gentle undulations, and small octopuses that on being disturbed discharge a brilliant purple, ink-like, fluid as a sort of smoke-screen. And there is also an amazing diversity of sea-anemones, starfish and crabs, and clams with corrugated mantles of bright blues, purples, greens, and browns. It was this commingled variety of colours of all these creatures that astonished me most, and I find it difficult to understand the reason for such a polychromatic display. They are all intermixed in close community with each other, occupying the same local habitat and apparently identical in their way of living and their demands on their immediate environment. I could not see that all this difference of colour served any direct function for the individual colonies of corals themselves, or, for that matter, for the clams and anemones and starfish and nudibranchs. I do not know that any satisfactory solution of this problem has ever been offered. I was reminded of the same conundrum later in my tour of Australia when I visited Perth in the spring-time and, exploring the surrounding country, marvelled at the multitude of different-coloured wild flowers all crowded together in the same limited territory. It may be that the colorations, at least some of them, are simply the by-products of different metabolic processes—like the hidden red of the haemoglobin of our blood corpuscles, or the bright yellows of fat, or the green of the bile within the human body, primarily serving no protective or attractive or other function that plays any part in the perpetuation of each species by natural selection. Or it may be that the kaleidoscopic intensity of the colours by their diversity and dazzling contrast in some way benefits the community as a whole.

Apart from my wanderings through the pools of the coral reef at low tide, I spent much of my time on the island sunbathing on the soft white sand and lazily watching the terns, gulls and shearwaters that gathered nearby. The water was pleasantly warm at midday and deliciously cold in the early morning for bathing. While it was the splendour of the sunsets in Borneo that I contemplated with such wonder, on the coral island it was the spreading radiance of the sunrise that particularly delighted me. At this hour of daybreak the opalescent tints of the eastern sky wove a most delicate pattern of the lightest yellows and pinks and soft greens that blended with the blue of the lightening sky.

It will probably be agreed that one of the benefits to be gained from staying on a small island is the purely psychological effect of an interval of isolation and solitude. But opinions will differ on the truth of such a surmise, varying with the natural temperament of each individual. Poets have from time to time praised the advantages of solitude. Byron puts the seeming paradox that 'In solitude we are *least* alone', but I think Milton emphasized the most reasonable argument in favour of a solitary retreat when he wrote in *Paradise Lost*, 'For solitude sometimes is best society—And short retirement urges sweet return.' I myself have frequently felt in the mood for temporary solitude. It is not that I am an unsociable sort of person; I have always enjoyed conversation among those with whom I have common interests and a common background, and—particularly as I advance in age—with old friends of many years' standing. Reminiscences of early days bring solace when one's active life begins to proceed gradually towards its inevitable close. But I confess I have never found it easy to engage wholeheartedly in what is sometimes called table-talk or chit-chat; I am temperamentally uneasy whenever I have to *make* conversation on matters that seem to me to be of trivial importance. Solitude and quietness provide the opportunity for meditation free from distractions, and for me the necessary occasion for sorting out personal difficulties and anxieties, and ordering complexities of mind into their proper perspective. Relief from disquietudes and responsibilities associated with the routine of a busy life not uncommonly leads on to solutions of problems that had previously seemed intractable. Occasions for meditative and constructive reflection may sometimes be provided by an island retreat. More commonly I have found such relief in a solitary walking holiday or scrambling up mountains—especially scrambling up mountains.

I am not in the least sense a 'mountaineer', but I think some of the moments when I have experienced my most exalted feelings of happiness have been on reaching the top of a mountain after the physical effort of clambering up to it on my own. I suppose this results, in part, from the sheer sense of achievement after contending with the difficulties and drudgery of a laborious ascent. Particularly is this the case when one has had to battle with unforeseen obstacles, or unexpected hazards of rain or snow or mist. But I have a poor head for heights, and during a climb up Tryfan from Lake Ogwen in a swirling mist that exaggerated the craggy precipices out of all proportion to their reality, there were points of the ascent that really terrified me. I must confess to a similar feeling of apprehension when, after climbing up the steep eastern slope of Crib Goch covered with winter snow, I traversed some quite narrow stretches of the ridge leading to the top of Snowdon, a climb which to a mountaineer would be regarded as no more than a mountain ramble. Such excursions among the Welsh mountains, alarming to me when I had to edge my way along the margin of a precipice or negotiate steeply sloping screes, are now more pleasurable in retrospect because one tends to forget the moments of trepidation or to remember them only as thrills of expectation and achievement, as indeed they were. Some of the mountains of the Lake District offer similar hazards, and to be suddenly enshrouded in one of the thick mists that may abruptly descend on them as happened to me on a memorable occasion can give rise to moments of trepidation even if you are well supplied with compass and maps.

Climbing mountains in Borneo may be more arduous because of the wet, slippery tracks of the rain forest, but at least their trees and creepers usually provide plenty of handgrips in support of precarious footholds. During my three years in Sarawak I only had opportunities for climbing some of the lesser mountains, a pity because the more elevated heights offered particularly exciting prospects of novel scenery. Reaching the top of the Matang range was rewarding because of the panoramic view of lowland forests extending for miles over Sarawak on the one side and on the other of what was then called Dutch Borneo. And I once climbed alone the mountain at the entry of the Kuching river, Santubong, which was fairly easy going until I neared the summit where its steepness approaches verticality. But descending again was simple and rather unusual, for without making very much use of my feet I swung myself down arm over arm from the close-packed tree trunks and their branches, an exhilarating mode of travel. As I remember, I thought at the time that I was temporarily reverting atavistically to a very primitive kind of locomotion, one that has been highly developed by the anthropoid apes of today with their long clinging arms—a method of progression that is called brachiation. In fact, I was for a time a brachiating Primate, and very lively I found this descent to be. Santubong is an impressive mountain though not very high—rather less than three thousand feet—and it stands up like a massive bastion protecting the entrance to the river. It had become curiously related in a legendary reference to the first Rajah of Sarawak. The mountain is visible from the town of Kuching some miles away and from here it projects on the northern horizon as a dominating feature of the landscape. From this view-point the uneven contour of its eastern slopes bears a singular resemblance to a silhouette of the face of Sir James Brooke, and in days gone past this was regarded by the local Malays as more than a fortuitous resemblance; it was taken to be a natural symbol of the initiation of the Brooke rule that liberated the people of Sarawak from the evil times of piracy and hardship which preceded the proclamation of the first White Rajah in 1841.

If you look down from a mountain top to a river winding its unceasing flow far down in a valley below, you will perhaps be struck by the seeming incongruity between them. The stability and immobility of the mountain contrasts so strongly with the restless flurryings of the river. The one gives the impression of unchanging permanence, the other of unrelated and evanescent fluctuation. Yet the reverse is the case. Rivers commonly owe their very existence to mountains where streams converge into rivulets and these into the main rivers themselves. And in many cases mountains owe their origin to rivers that carve out deep valleys or gorges from what many ages ago was a high plateau, leaving behind them isolated relics of the latter still reaching up to the clouds. The valleys are, so to speak, negative images of the mountains, and it is rather the mountains that are evanescent features eventually to be eroded and flattened by the disintegrating forces of water action, while the rivers continue their onward flow. But, after all, the whole process is a relative one, for even rivers are not immutable—their levels change with the passage of time, their course may be altered by geological events, and with increasing aridity they may dry up and disappear altogether.

I find that I have always tended, subconsciously perhaps, to relate different periods of life to the rivers and streams associated with them. The first river that consciously occupied my mind when I was about seven years old was the Severn at Newnham where my father was for a short period the vicar, and I think it was the appearance of its irresistible flow, accelerated at regular intervals by an imposing and rather sinister-looking bore plunging up towards Gloucester, that brought to full consciousness that particular dimension of experience which we call 'time'. It is common enough, of course, for time to be compared with the flow of water—'Time like an ever-rolling stream', 'Time's fleeting river' and so forth. But to the child's mind the unremitting flow of time is not at first apparent—the small world in which he lives seems to be almost static. Certain changes are indeed apparent, from day to night, from summer to winter, and from one birthday to another. But these appear as cyclic changes merely repeating themselves, and the stretching out of the future is as yet unperceived. It was then or perhaps a little later, I forget exactly when, that the fancy presented itself to me quite naturally that if time is really like an ever-rolling stream, then in our journey through life it is as though we are rowing in a boat with our face towards the stern, watching the receding series of events of the past, but without being able to turn round and view clearly the details of our future course. By oblique glances over the shoulder we may catch vague glimpses out of the corner of the eye and thus get some general indication of the direction in which we should guide ourselves, but there can be no certain predictability of the future.

When I was nine years old my mother died and it was this that decided my father to leave Newnham. Thus we moved from Gloucestershire to Devon, from the valley of the Severn to the valley of the Exe, my father having been appointed the rector of a tiny village near Tiverton called Washfield. A mile or two away was a tributary of the river Exe, here narrowed

and made the more exciting by the damming up of a local
tributary to form a cascading weir. I used to bathe regularly in
the river with my brothers during the summer, though when it
was in full spate after heavy rains, transforming itself from what
was little more than a placid stream into a torrential river, it
called for a little daring even for a reasonably good swimmer.
I joined my brothers at Blundell's School in 1910 after leaving
The Wells House, a preparatory school at Malvern Wells, and
at the age of seventeen I started my career as a medical student
in October 1912. This next stage of my life I associate with
two rivers, in term time the Thames flowing alongside the
terrace of St. Thomas's Hospital, and the Teign in south Devon
during vacations (for by now my father had moved once again,
this time to retirement at Teignmouth). In ruminating
retrospectively over this period, time seems to have carried me
forward in a wider and ever more swiftly flowing current.
Earlier remembered experiences of childhood stand out as little
trickles isolated from each other in a nebulous landscape of
vaguely remembered routine. Later experiences converge
more and more completely into swelling tributaries that
finally empty into a broad and continuous stream of conscious
realization. Odd and apparently unconnected items of knowledge acquired here and there in youth begin to interweave and
coalesce one with another, and in acquiring cohesion become
more coherent. A plan of existence then seems dimly to be
perceived and evokes the need for a general plan of action to
give effect to personal aspirations. It is thus that each one of us
develops for himself his own philosophy of life and living—a
philosophy that may broadly correspond with that of his fellows
but is never completely coincident in all its details.

During our holidays at Teignmouth, my two brothers and I
used to go on walking tours from time to time, usually over
Dartmoor or Exmoor. On one occasion we decided to walk,
over a matter of several days, from the source of the river

Teign to its terminal estuary. We aimed to start with Cranmere Pool which is hidden in the very centre of Dartmoor and was commonly said—not quite correctly—to mark the actual beginning of the Teign. It was also reported to be very difficult to find. In fact we did not find it, for starting out from Chagford one day and having crossed Watern Tor on to Taw Head, we were rather suddenly enveloped in one of the Dartmoor mists that have a habit of appearing with little warning. We therefore decided to turn back because, although we had compasses to direct us, we were uncertain of the where-abouts of bogs and marshy areas that may be quite treacherous in such weather (I always associate these Dartmoor explorations with Conan Doyle's novel *The Hound of the Baskervilles* and the climax of Grimpen Mire that I had read about this time). However, we did start down river at Teign Head close by and followed what was no more than a mountain stream babbling its descent past Sittaford Tor, past stone circles, and past the wooded valley of Gidleigh with its remnants of a fourteenth century castle. Then on through the old market town of Chagford where the mountain rivulet had begun to earn the more dignified title of a river, having been joined by the South Teign tributary that starts as a spring of water near the stone circles of Grey Wethers. From Chagford the Teign runs eastwards and cuts its way through the picturesque gorge of Fingle, dominated on one side by Prestonbury Hill topped by the earthworks of an ancient camp and crossed below by the weathered stone arches of Fingle Bridge. Lower down, the river turns south and gains a more sophisticated air by joining company with the railway that runs alongside it to Chudleigh. About three miles south of this small town the Teign is joined by the Bovey river, and, broadening out, runs at a more gentle tempo through the lower ground of a wider valley. We also explored the course of the Bovey river; this rises near the middle of Dartmoor not far from the origin of the South

Teign tributary, passes the little village of North Bovey and, gathering momentum as it descends to lower levels over faulted rocky strata, cuts through Lustleigh Cleave for about two miles. The steep side of the Cleave valley is strewn here and there with mighty rocks of granite rolled down, I suppose, by torrents in the long ago erosion of what was a high plateau of Dartmoor. It is the odd remnants of this extinct plateau that have been left behind to form the characteristic tors of Dartmoor. And now down through Bovey Tracey overlooked by the humpy skyline of Haytor. From here the course of the Teign is aligned parallel with railway and main road and begins to acquire a certain artificiality as it approaches the urban civilization represented by the unattractive town of Newton Abbot. Thereafter it broadens out suddenly to a width of a quarter of a mile or so, forming a tidal estuary that extends directly to Teignmouth four miles away. This last part of the journey down the Teign in our young days was particularly pleasant—the road traffic was scanty then, and it was even more pleasant when we made a slight detour over the southern slopes of Haldon Moor because of the splendid view of rounded hills over the opposite side of the valley, tesseleated with a patchwork of green fields. And finally to the mouth of the river, once a harbour of some importance but less so now that its entrance to the sea is to a large extent hemmed in by a sand-bank. Its narrowed exit is dominated by the impressive mass of red sandstone called the Ness, overlaid by a coverlet of trees and fringed at its base by a scattering of huge boulders hurled down by past erosion and subsidence of the cliff face.

I have given this brief description of one of our many walking tours partly to commend to those who enjoy walking the stimulating idea of exploring a river from its initial source in a mountain spring to its grand finale where it enters the sea. In following its course thus, a river comes to be seen, not as a local stretch of water that by itself may appear almost mono-

CPE R

tonous in its uniformity, but as an organized and lively system which has gradually been developed by the synthesis of a multitude of contributing rivulets struggling over obstacles of geological unconformities, boring their way through rock and soil and carving out valleys, until at last they converge into the main stream. So, again, one is led to look back and consider the genesis and geological history of the river in past ages and to look forward to envisage the unceasing changes that must inexorably continue to alter its contour and configuration in future ages. By analogy, as I have earlier remarked, we look back on our own life and recognize how momentarily detached experiences, and isolated springs of knowledge acquired here and there, finally flow together to constitute the essence of a full-grown personality. Only there is this difference; the onward course of an individual life never reaches the ultimate calm of an open sea—it is like a never-ending river which has perpetually to contend with and adjust itself to never-ending changes.

A river may sometimes digress from what seems to be the more direct course it should naturally take towards its destination, perhaps the result of local variations of landscape. And here I shall allow myself a page or two of digression in order briefly to recall the happy days of our walking tours in Devonshire. We took these journeys seriously in our exploration of the country through which we travelled, but we delighted in them physically as well as sensuously. We walked ourselves hard in all weathers, and stayed frugally at little cottages wherever, on arrival at our temporary destination, we could find accommodation with bed and breakfast for about four or five shillings for each of us. We thoroughly enjoyed ourselves and found plenty of occasion for hilarity. They were joyous days those, days of conviviality and close comradeship. I was the youngest of us three. My eldest brother Bill was then an undergraduate at Balliol College where he had gained a scholarship and was reading 'Greats'. Parenthetically, I should mention that his real name is not Bill—it is a nickname he acquired and has retained ever since the First World War when in the ranks he grew a somewhat untidy moustache that drew a comparison with Bruce Bairnsfather's famous caricature of 'Old Bill'. I think it is true to say that he had the most acute intellect of us all. He was possessed of an unusually seeking and searching mind and cast his attention far and wide beyond the immediate requirements of his university subjects at Oxford, delving into philosophy, psychology, biological and physical sciences, literature, history ancient and modern, and many other fields of learning. He had not only a very receptive mentality but also a very retentive one, and his powers of memorization seemed to me to be phenomenal. Thus later on, with his encyclopaedic knowledge cultivated in depth as well as in width, he was well able to hold his own in argumentative discussions with recognized authorities in many diverse branches of scholarship. Naturally enough he picked my brains each time I returned home on vacation from my medical school in London so as to imbibe in theory much that I had learnt in practice. More than that, he wanted personally on one ocasion to examine and dissect a human brain for himself because of his interest in current work in psychology, and for this purpose he persuaded me to bring one home from St. Thomas's Hospital preserved in formalin. I remember feeling a touch of guilt in doing so, for it was strictly against regulations, and also quite illegal, to remove any part of a human body from the dissecting room of the medical school. I particularly recollect travelling down by train from Paddington to Teignmouth with the human brain tied up in a brown paper parcel on the rack, and wondering to myself what the elderly lady sitting beneath it would think if she knew what the parcel contained. We systematically dissected that brain in an attic room behind locked doors, feeling much as the early anatomists

CPE R*

of Vesalius' time must have felt when they had secretly to make their anatomical studies on corpses because of the religious proscription on the dissection of human bodies.

My second brother, Cyril, was essentially a practical man, a man of action, more so than either Bill or myself at that time. Like us, he was intensely interested in natural history, but more in field work than in speculative enquiries. For example, while we on occasion engaged ourselves in the sort of bird study related more to the academic side of ornithology, Cyril was rather the 'bird watcher'. While we were interested in the structure and classification of birds, in their evolutionary history, in their protective coloration and sexual display, or in the various theories put forward to account for the curious phenomena of bird migration, he was better acquainted with local bird life and more adept at spotting and identifying the different kinds of birds that we saw on our walks. While we sought in the current literature for explanations of the differences in colour and shape of bird's eggs, he made a fine collection of them by his greater facility in locating birds' nests. But there was another facet in his attitude of mind during our under-graduate days, aroused I think by the publication some years earlier of a book by Erskine Childers entitled *The Riddle of the Sands*, which in the form of a novel recounted secret service and espionage activities in the North Sea area and presaged the possibility of an invasion of England by the Germans. Cyril took this seriously and developed a political consciousness which we, with our many interests in other directions, perhaps tended to overlook. So, when in exploring the country around Bill and I sought to interpret the various features of the landscape in terms of geological formations, surface erosions, weathering, climatic fluctuations in past ages and so forth, Cyril tended to look at them in terms of military strategy. Not that he was in any sense a 'militarist', but I think he vaguely apprehended the looming ahead of international conflict even if he did not at the time formulate in his mind any specific details of what this conflict might involve. But he was certainly endowed with great intellectual ability, though this was for the time lying latent or subordinated to interests of more immediately practical import. He displayed his gift of scholarship much later in life when he was engaged on duties in the Far East. For it was while at Amoy that, in an astonishingly short time, he acquired so intimate an acquaintance with the Chinese language that he published a unique and fully annotated translation of an eleventh-century Chinese poet, Su Tung-P'o. A distinguished sinologist, Dr Gustav Ecke, was moved to comment that the notes and commentaries accompanying the translation testified to a profound learning and also showed a most congenial feeling for the very spirit of Chinese civilisation. 'This work', he went on to say, 'will remain as one of the outstanding Western contributions to the study of Chinese literature.'

As I have already tried to indicate, we had no occasion in our Teignmouth days for recognizing Cyril's purely intellectual potentialities; he was then too concerned in his mind with the current trend of world affairs. But the interests of all three of us, though each having their own particularity, ran parallel and at their margins overlapped and intermingled, tending always to stream out into a tide of common interest. It was at the end of one of our walking tours over Dartmoor that the declaration of war on 4 August 1914 was announced. I have a vivid memory of that expedition when on reaching home we crossed the estuary of the Teign by ferry boat from Shaldon to Teignmouth. Like many people we persuaded ourselves that the war would be sharp and short (with our side the victors, naturally), and like many others we were caught up in the general excitement of the time. We could not foresee, nor did we ever imagine, the tragedies that would follow, nor did it occur to us that this was to be the last time we three would ever again be able to renew the delights of our walking tours.

While it is true to say that Borneo is predominantly a land of forest and jungle that impede easy communications between its different geographical areas, it is equally true to say that it is a land of rivers that facilitate these communications. In 1920 when I went to Sarawak to take up my post as Principal Medical Officer there were no main roads linking up one Division of the country with another. Thus, in travelling to inland villages and outstations, rivers were our main highways, and it was commonly necessary to go downstream by river, along the coast by sea, and upstream by another river to reach our destination. Today the situation is very different, for with the rapid growth of the population over the last forty years the need has arisen for the intensive development of Sarawak agriculturally and commercially in an attempt to make it more self-supporting, and interconnecting roads between the main Divisions of the country have become of increasing importance.

There were some of my colleagues in Sarawak who seemed to find the slow journeys in motor launches along the lower stretches of the main rivers tedious and uninteresting because the scenery for miles was often monotonous. For myself these river expeditions suited my mood at the time. They gave me leisure for contemplation in a spirit of mental relaxation, and I welcomed the occasional pleasant interludes in my medical and administrative duties during which I could prepare plans for developing medical centres that I was on my way to visit, or consider how best to deal with problems in the medical centres from which I was returning. From this point of view the rivers were not really interruptions of my administrative duties, they were an essential part of them. But I also found them interesting interludes, for in their lower reaches the rivers were continually on the twist and turn through immense tracts of lowland jungle, so that I always seemed to be about to turn a corner with the inevitable curiosity of seeing what would be revealed beyond it.

On reaching shallower water at higher levels it was necessary to transfer from launch to a 'prahu' manned by Dyaks with their paddles. The scenery now became more variegated, and the river banks strewn with pebbles and water-worn boulders. And at intervals we had to navigate our craft over a series of rapids. Shooting these rapids in downward journey is an exciting experience, and I always marvelled at the incredible skill of the Dyaks when manoeuvring the prahu in a zig-zag course among huge rocks between which the channels of water swirled and cascaded. It was once while shooting such a rapid that I acquired quite an undeserved reputation as a 'crack shot'. I used to carry with me on these excursions up-country a small ·22 rifle for collecting purposes should I see a rare creature that I might want to study, and on this particular occasion I saw a crocodile lying on the top of a rock basking asleep in the sun. I took hurried aim as we swept past and by an extraordinary fluke I suppose I must have hit the animal in what is said to be its most vulnerable spot—in the soft under-skin near the base of the foreleg. At any rate it curled up backwards in a sudden spasm, turned a somersault, and fell apparently dead into the water. The spurious prestige as a marksman that I thus gained aroused much admiration from my Dyak crew, to the extent that I found it very difficult to convince them that it was no more than a chance shot.

No doubt my most pleasant recollections of Sarawak rivers are those of the tidal river of Kuching. From time to time in the evening as a means of relaxation I used to paddle restfully up the river in my small sampan. Going upstream I kept in view the Matang mountain range, beginning to be crowned with sunset clouds that gradually reddened centripetally from their margins into a fiery incandescence. I think I have never seen such a succession of glorious sunsets as those which were to be seen over Matang; it would be useless for me to try to describe them in words, for words could not possibly convey the wonder of their splendour. After sunset when the sky was overcome by its rapid darkening I would turn and paddle back to Kuching in the light of the moon and stars. It was serenely peaceful and quiet except for the ripple of the water, the strokes of my paddle, and maybe in the distance the seductive cadences of a Malay youth singing in plaintive pentatonic melody a love song. And when darkness had grown almost to completion, the fireflies would light up in the branches of the sonneratia trees along the river bank, sparkling and flickering, sometimes seeming to flash in rhythmic unison, and outshining the distant stars by the concentrated brilliance of their scintillations.

After my return from Borneo in 1923 rivers came to form a rather indistinct background to pressing matters of academic and domestic life, though they continued to excite my imagination in many ways. There was the little tributary of the River Lee by our home in Digswell with the biblical-sounding name of the Mimram, an appropriate name derived from an Anglo-Saxon term meaning a babbling brook. At Oxford I at first found myself perplexed by its confusing entanglement of rivers and canals, so confusing that even now, after many years, I have to think a few moments before I can identify by name a particular water way. And now, as I write, I look down on the Valley of the Evenlode, a small homely river meandering its way along a broad valley out of all proportion in its width. Here you can wander by footpaths through fields and copses along its unfrequented and winding course, following the movements of its moorhens, mallards, swans, kingfishers and water-rats, admiring its irises, bulrushes, water-lilies, and its banks multicoloured with wild flowers, and watching the tresses of vivid green weeds that wave languidly in its currents (that somehow always remind me of Millais' painting of

Ophelia). Hilaire Belloc in his 'Dedicatory Ode' wrote of the Evenlode as

> A lovely river, all alone
> She lingers in the hills and holds
> A hundred little towns of stone
> Forgotten in the western wolds.

And that is how it appears to me.

In this chapter I have let my pen wander on to islands, up mountains, and along rivers. What I have recounted in these meditations are some of the incidents that tend to isolate themselves from a continuity of diverse experiences simply because they are particularly happy phrases of melody in what Walt Whitman has expressed as a 'chant of pleasant exploration'. Adventures of this sort surge up from time to time into conscious recollection as later years go by, giving inspiration in the routine duties of day-to-day life, and sometimes solace in the moods of depression that sporadically affect most of us when we need to face difficulties and disappointments.

It is good that the lapse of time tends to dull the less pleasant experiences of the past and to high-light the more pleasant. Those moments of hard tragedy that most of us of older years have experienced, particularly those who have been involved in two World Wars, are for ever vivid in the memory, and there also remain nagging reminders of long and troublesome efforts that have met with frustration and disillusionment. By and large, however, difficulties and discomforts do tend to be forgotten—outshone, as it were, by occasional successes that interrupt them. At the time of their occurrence physical or mental exertion may be accompanied by unpleasant sensations of fatigue and exhaustion, perhaps reaching near the limits of tolerance in the strain which they impose. But, paradoxically as it may appear, if the exertions culminate in the fulfilment of a longed-for objective, the toil and drudgery are remembered retrospectively as enjoyable experiences because they somehow become merged indistinguishably with the happiness occasioned by the final achievement.

At any rate, I myself have found it to be thus.

Printed by Robert Cunningham & Sons Ltd, Alva